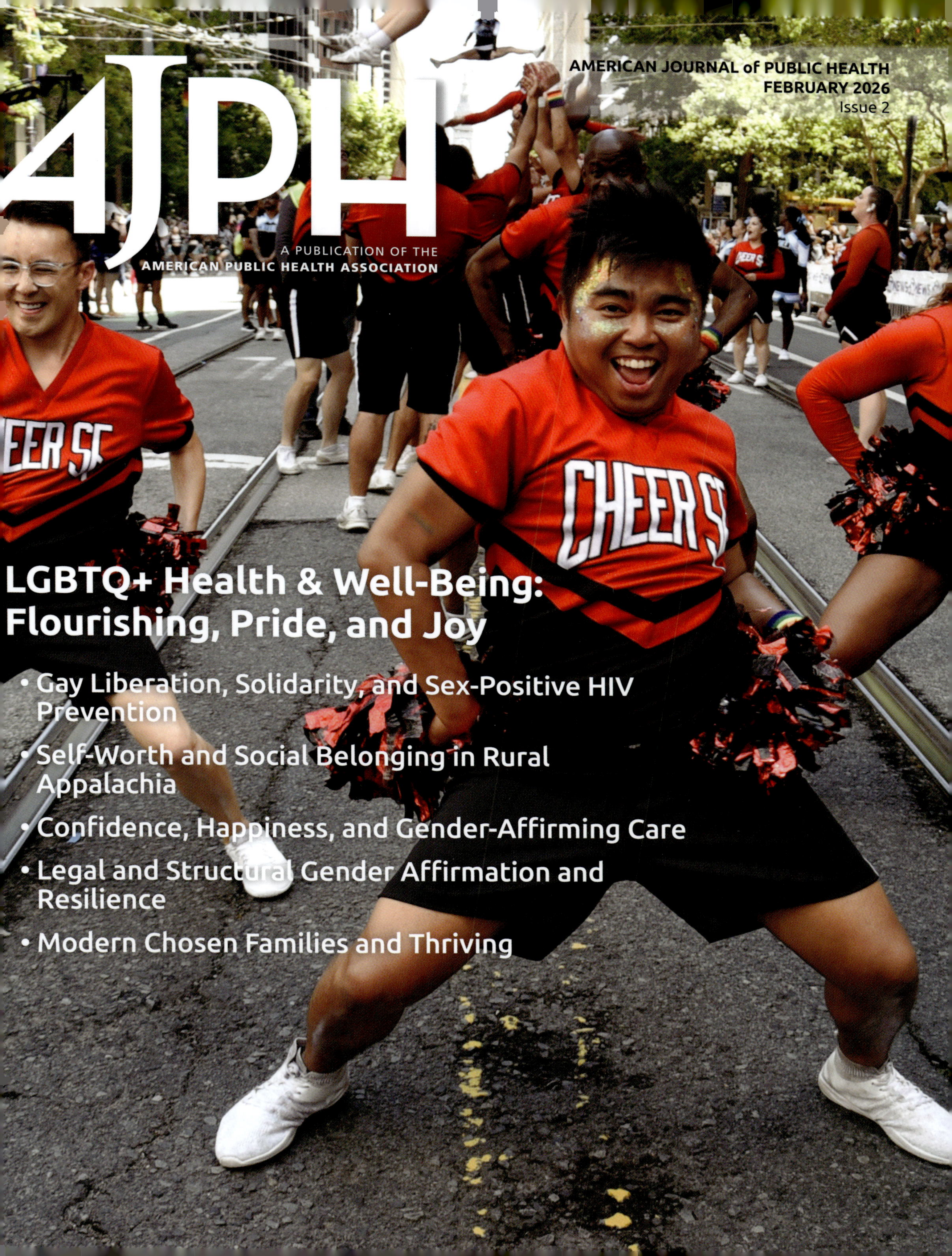

AJPH

A PUBLICATION OF THE
AMERICAN PUBLIC HEALTH ASSOCIATION

AMERICAN JOURNAL of PUBLIC HEALTH
FEBRUARY 2026
Issue 2

LGBTQ+ Health & Well-Being: Flourishing, Pride, and Joy

- Gay Liberation, Solidarity, and Sex-Positive HIV Prevention
- Self-Worth and Social Belonging in Rural Appalachia
- Confidence, Happiness, and Gender-Affirming Care
- Legal and Structural Gender Affirmation and Resilience
- Modern Chosen Families and Thriving

AJPH®, published monthly, is the official Journal of the American Public Health Association®, 800 I St NW, Washington, DC 20001-3710; (202) 777- APHA; TDD (202) 777-2500. APHA is a nongovernmental professional society founded in 1872, representing all disciplines and specialties in public health.

The *American Journal of Public Health*® (*AJPH*) (print ISSN: 0090-0036; electronic ISSN: 1541- 0048), first published in 1911, is the official journal of the American Public Health Association® (APHA). The oldest and largest organization of public health professionals in the world, APHA represents approximately 30 000 members from more than 50 occupations of public health.

Submissions: Visit www.editorialmanager.com/ajph for online manuscript preparation and submission guidelines. Contributions of original unpublished research, social science analyses, scholarly essays, critical commentaries, departments, and letters to the editor are welcome. Questions? Write ajph.submissions@apha.org or call APHA at (202) 777-2469.

Print plus online subscriptions: Institutional price (print copy with online access) for a single institution and all authorized users, regardless of geographic location varies by size of organization; multiple campuses not permitted without special arrangement. To order, write apha.subscriptions@apha.org.

Online-only subscriptions: Institutional price for one US federal institution and its authorized users is $1,015–$1,510. To order, write apha.subscriptions@apha.org. For academic, non-US federal consortia, or multisite subscriptions, contact apha.subscriptions@apha.org or visit http://research.ebsco.com for pricing information.

Print-only subscriptions: Institutional price is US $970, $1,065 international.

Back print issues: A limited number of print issues are for sale. Single copies are US $80, $90 international (air delivery). Shipping and handling fees will apply; prepay only. To order, write apha.subscriptions@apha.org.

Reprints: For prices and ordering information on 50 or more reprints, check the Reprints section at www.ajph.org. To order smaller quantities of reprints (rush delivery), use the "Purchase Article" link on the article site itself.

Electronic access: Online articles more than 10 years old are available free for personal use at www.ajph.org. Recent articles are available through pay-per-view: single PDF article for $24, single issue access for 24 hours for $33, or entire site access for 24 hours for $38.

Postal information: Periodicals postage paid at Washington, DC, and additional mailing offices. Postmaster: Send address changes to American Journal of Public Health, 800 I St NW, Washington, DC 20001-3710.

Address changes: Send to AJPH, Membership Department (members) or AJPH Subscriptions (subscribers), APHA, 800 I St NW, Washington, DC 20001-3710. Or write to membership.mail@apha.org (members) or apha.subscriptions@apha.org (subscribers).

Indexes: Publications that index or abstract articles from *AJPH* include the following: Ageline, Assia (Applied Social Science Index and Abstracts), Biological Abstracts, Chemical Abstracts, CINAHL, Criminal Justice Abstracts, EMBASE, EMCare, Environmental Abstracts, e-psyche, ERIC, ETOH (Alcohol and Alcohol Problems Science Database), Excerpta Medica, Food Science and Technology, General Science Index, Grateful Med, Hospital Literature Index, Human Resources Abstracts, International Pharmaceutical Abstracts (IPA), Medline, Physical Education Index, Pollution Abstracts, Psychological Abstracts, PsychINFO, Safety Science Abstracts, Sage Family Studies Abstracts, Sage Human Resources Abstracts, Science Citation Index, SCOPUS, SIIC Data Bases, Social Work Research and Abstracts, and Statistical Reference Index (SRI)/LexisNexis.

AJPH
A PUBLICATION OF THE
AMERICAN PUBLIC HEALTH ASSOCIATION

COVER: Local cheer groups perform during the Gay Pride Parade on June 29, 2025, in San Francisco, California.

Cover concept and selection by Aleisha Kropf. Photo by Meera Fox/Getty Images. Printed with permission.

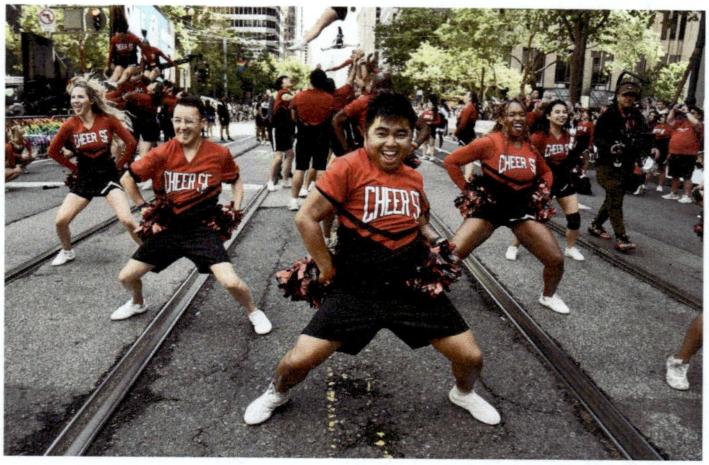

APHA
AMERICAN PUBLIC HEALTH ASSOCIATION
For science. For action. For health.

Promoting public health research, policy, practice, and education is the *AJPH* mission. As we widen our scope to embrace global issues, we also sharpen our focus to support the needs of public health practitioners. We invite contributions of original unpublished research, opinion and commentary, and letters to the editor.

The *Journal* is printed on acid-free recycled paper.

OPEN ACCESS   ONLINE ONLY   PODCAST   DATA SUPPLEMENT AVAILABLE

EDITOR'S CHOICE

157 Science in Service: Reflections on the MacArthur "Genius" Fellowship
N. Dasgupta

OPINIONS, IDEAS, & PRACTICE

EDITORIALS

159 LGBTQ Public Health Is Public Health: Advancing Equity When Institutions Falter
P. N. Halkitis and K. D. Krause

162 Short- and Long-Term Potential Impacts of Ongoing and Escalating Legal and Political Attacks on LGBTQ Health and Health Equity
D. Zubizarreta and A. L. Beccia

166 The Urgent Need for Evidence and Action on Global Transgender Mental Health
A. I. Scheim

168 How Political Dynamics May Shape Availability and Utilization of Health Care Services Through Federally Qualified Health Centers
E. K. Lee and M. B. Cole

171 Disaster Within a Disaster: Ensuring Access to Opioid Use Disorder Treatment During Natural Crises
E. Cerceo, C. Stearns, K. Shapley-Quinn, and M. Salzman

NOTES FROM THE FIELD

175 Roadblocks to Rural Health: State Transportation Policies' Impact on Health Care Access in Virginia's Rural Communities: 2021–2022
K. Y. Tossas, B. D. Owens, M. O'Grady, J. Zhao, and R. A. Winn

DISCUSSION

180 Reassessing Medicaid's Protective Effect During Continuous-Coverage Unwinding: A Focused Reanalysis and Practice Note
S. Zeng, S. Huang, W. Chen, and R. Li

182 Use of an Inappropriate Control Period When Exploring the Impacts of Cannabis Legalization
B. P. Smyth and P. McCarron

183 Myran et al. Respond
D. T. Myran, R. Pacula, and M. Taljaard

185 Reconsidering Conservative Exclusion Criteria in Claims-Based Research on Gender-Affirming Surgery
R. Sanaeikia

186 Babbs et al. Respond
G. Babbs, D. Dai, E. R. Boskey, E. Balkan, and J. M. W. Hughto

LGBTQ+ WELL-BEING & JOY

188 The Need to Focus on Flourishing LGBTQ+ Futures
B. E. Coston and S. Landers

192 Dangers of a Politically Motivated Research Agenda on Transgender Health
T. E. Schall, J. D. Moses, E. A. Dietz, L. E. Stamm, J. Penny, and A. I. Scheim

197 Flourishing Families: Promoting Public Health and Reproductive Justice for All by Protecting and Supporting LGBTQ+ Families in Policy and Practice
S. Mackenzie, N. N. Johnson, J. E. Scheib, L. Kali, and J. Wilson

202 Celebrating the Legacy and Urgency of Sex-Positive, Queer-Led Public Health
S. D. Rhodes

205 "It Has Transformed Living for Me": The Trajectory of Alignment, Comfort, and Social Connectedness After Gender-Affirming Surgery
T. Gaedecke, K. Jackman, M. George, M. Ryvicker, and W. Bockting

210 Transgender Youth Health and Joy: A Model of Evidence-Based School District Policy Change to Support Transgender and Nonbinary Youth Health
S. Mackenzie, N. Mann, and O. Hertenstein

RESEARCH & ANALYSIS

LGBTQ+ WELL-BEING & JOY

214 Sex-Positive HIV Prevention Messages: A Case Study From the Early Years of the Epidemic
C. W. Adrian, S. G. Massey, J. B. Haager, and E. Lowinger

222 Unconventional Resilience: Necessary Social Identity Management Among Asylum-Seeking Sexual and Gender-Diverse Survival Migrants
D. C. Agor, C. Nnaji, C. Alvarez, J. Bauermeister, and S. Meanley

229 Association Between Gender Affirmation and Adoption Interest Among a Large Sample of Transgender, Nonbinary, and Gender-Diverse Populations in Washington State, 2023
A. Ogunbajo, T. DeAtley, A. Breslow, K. Gamarel, D. Operario, T. Kershaw, R. L. E. Tavernier, and A. J. Restar

240 Structural Cissexism, Mental Health, and Unmet Health Care Needs Among Gender-Diverse Adolescents in the United States
H. Lee, T. R. Sullivan, J. R. Abramson, P. S. McCauley, R. J. Watson, and E. H. Mereish

OPEN-THEMED RESEARCH

251 Evaluation of a Novel Data Source for National Influenza Surveillance: Influenza Hospitalization Data in the National Healthcare Safety Network, United States, September 2021–April 2024
A. M. Frutos, S. Moon, A. M. Binder, A. J. Cool, K. Iyawe, T. Thompson, M. A. Dudeck, C. H. Bozio, M. W. Tenforde, M. Biggerstaff, and K. M. Sumner

256 Contextualizing President Trump's Executive Orders Targeting Transgender Health and Gender-Affirming Care
N. Nuruzzaman and E. Hsiang

261 Association of Discrimination and Violence With Suicidality Among *Travestis* and Transgender Women in Rio de Janeiro, Brazil, 2015–2023: A Cross-Sectional Study
D. R. A. Coelho, E. M. Jalil, B. Fernandes, E. Peixoto, T. Vianna, M. Ramos, C. M. Jalil, L. Ferreira, I. B. Moura, R. K. Friedman, A. C. Araujo, S. C. Wagner, S. L. Reisner, A. S. Keuroghlian, V. G. Veloso, B. Grinsztejn, and C. Coutinho

270 Political Boundaries, Health Care Gaps: The Link Between Gerrymandering and Federally Qualified Health Center Availability
A. E. Cote-L'Heureux and D. L. Chin

Science in Service: Reflections on the MacArthur "Genius" Fellowship

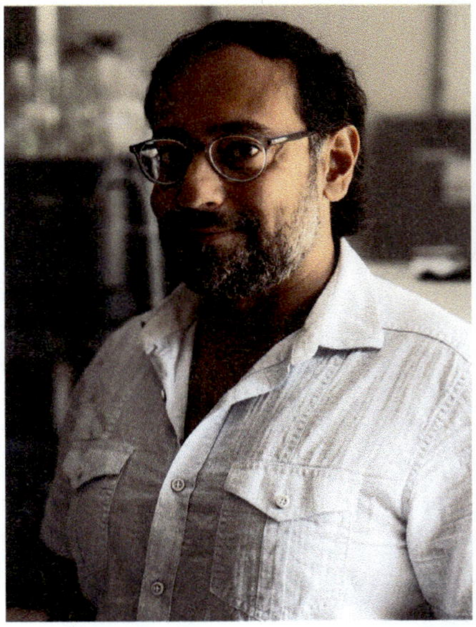

Nasbarun Dasgupta, PhD, MPH
Associate Editor, *AJPH*
Gillings School of Global Public Health, University of North Carolina at Chapel Hill
2025 MacArthur Fellow

At the American Public Health Association (APHA) annual meeting in November, speakers repeatedly described public health as the "invisible shield" protecting US communities. In side conversations outside the formal sessions, I heard a more personal resonance: many practitioners felt the phrase applied to them as well. They, too, feel invisible.

It is easy to understand why. Lists of verboten words circulate. Layoffs mount, and vital roles are labeled "nonessential." Massive multidisciplinary projects and data sets vanish. Career scientists within government are silenced.

Yet, at the opening plenary of the 2025 APHA Annual Meeting and Expo, the organization's executive director, Georges Benjamin, noted that this moment coincides with "communication at the speed of electrons." Taken together, these conditions suggest a growing disconnect between who does the work and who receives the credit.

Well, I for one have received enough credit and adulation to last a lifetime. In October, I was selected for one of the 22 MacArthur Fellowships—often referred to as "genius grants"—for my work in overdose prevention. This prestigious award, spanning all aspects of society, comes with five years of unrestricted funding. Because the selection process is confidential, nobody applies, and nobody knows they are being considered. The committees spend more than a year reviewing candidates and gathering independent evaluations. To receive that improbable telephone call is a dream so sublime it defies expectation.

Only a handful of public health practitioners have received this award in its 45-year history (far fewer than biomedical scientists). In a highly collaborative field such as public health, the singular nature of the honor obscures the underlying nature of who does the hands-on work and caregiving. I have not packed the thousands of boxes of naloxone and drug-checking kits we distribute, nor am I the one who analyzes drug samples in the lab, nor do I conduct street outreach. The current decline in overdose deaths reflects the labor of extraordinarily dedicated team members and the hundreds of frontline workers who make public health happen every day.

When news of the award broke, I was immensely relieved to hear many in the harm reduction and public health communities describe it as a win for themselves and for the field as a whole, which it undoubtedly was. Never has appropriation felt so appropriate.

Sharing credit is one of the qualities that makes public health a distinctive profession. Another is that the work we do has immense social ramifications. We continue to show up for our jobs—yes for the paycheck but also because most of us find the work meaningful. In our microcommunities, we can see the effects of what we do: we have a sense of who did not get sick, who recovered, who is better off because of our efforts. We know the outbreaks we helped contain, the meals delivered, the contamination cleaned up.

Amid the daily tumult of logistics and reports and caregiving, we can lose sight of the incredible privilege of working in a profession devoted to social impact. Few in the profession are motivated by public recognition, yet positive reinforcement can be a salve for burnout: it helps counteract relegation and invisibility. Collectively, we call this way of working "science in service."

In this moment of disenfranchisement, it strikes me that, to keep doing the work, we must become better at showing our work. We must also speak up for those whose efforts are

AJPH February 2026, Vol. 116, No. 2

minimized or overlooked. Those of us operating with megaphones and independence—including patient advocates, people with lived experience representing their communities, extraordinary outreach workers, clinical staff, and federal officials under gag orders—can do more to amplify the voices of the marginalized.

We as public health practitioners should avail ourselves of more opportunities to articulate the work we do and why it matters for the greater good. This applies both to our individual contributions and to our collective efforts. Academic conferences are not enough. The humble double-sided pamphlet, professional social media, photo and video essays, community presentations, and news media engagement are attainable. And if you prefer not to be in front of the camera yourself, elevate a partner organization instead.

The objective is not ego-laden puffery. It is a responsibility to offer an authentic alternative narrative that showcases our impact: show our work to show our worth. Put another way, instead of reacting to the daily political opprobrium, we stand to benefit from crafting a creative and affirmative vision for health in the United States.

After the pandemic's overreaches and a decade of deepening bureaucratization, public health policy has come to be viewed in popular culture as shorthand for the worst excesses of big government. Yet most public health practice happens quietly, in the unglamorous, everyday work of community caregiving. As Eliza Wheeler of the nonprofit Remedy Alliance For The People exhorts us: "Celebrate a populist public health!"

Ancient wisdom teaches that it costs nothing to elevate others. This principle has driven my own work for the past two decades. In each group I have choosen to join, I have sought out this motivating mindset. Our time is finite, and we can choose to align ourselves with people who uphold our values; this is, I would argue, just as important as any enticing scientific credential, if not more so.

As our vocation demands, we must also look to the root causes of the credit mismatch. I have had the honor of speaking at state summits for those engaged in local overdose prevention efforts funded through opioid settlements. Looking out across the thousands of faces, I am struck by how many of the attendees are women. That credit does not flow for this painstaking work is not surprising, given the social tendency to devalue labor based on who performs it, including people with lived experience. Their strength is their persistence.
The hard-won gains in reversing the decades-long increase in overdose deaths have largely been through steadfast science-driven care. Across the country, I see neighbors taking care of neighbors, far removed from the macho national rhetoric about stopping drug shipments with walls, drones, or warships. In rural communities and urban clusters alike, nobody wise is waiting for airstrikes on boats in the Caribbean. Instead, we take care of our own.

Hear this: what you are doing is working. Keep going, and embrace the opportunity to elevate your successes. The stories that matter most unfold at the local level. We can draw on the meaning that keeps us moving through our daily duties, reclaim the narrative, and place credit where it belongs: with the people doing the caregiving. AJPH

DOI: https://doi.org/10.2105/AJPH.2025.308375

ORCID iD:
Nasbarun Dasgupta https://orcid.org/0000-0002-4098-605X

LGBTQ Public Health Is Public Health: Advancing Equity When Institutions Falter

Perry N. Halkitis, PhD, MS, MPH, and Kristen D. Krause, PhD, MPH

ABOUT THE AUTHORS

Perry N. Halkitis and Kristen D. Krause are with the School of Public Health, Rutgers University, Newark and Piscataway, NJ.

Public health is both a scientific and a profoundly human enterprise; it is anchored in evidence yet inseparable from compassion, justice, and the moral imperative to protect the most vulnerable. The story of lesbian, gay, bisexual, transgender, and queer (LGBTQ) public health and our own journeys as a cisgender gay man and queer woman illustrate this truth. Like our own scholarly trajectories, LGBTQ public health did not emerge through institutional generosity but through the insistence of communities demanding to be respected and to have access to competent and effective prevention and care.

Our history teaches that progress has never arrived by invitation. When we could not reveal our whole selves to our health care providers (a reality to this day),[1] and when our sexuality was deemed a psychological disorder,[2] LGBTQ people built systems of care for ourselves. The modern era of LGBTQ health was forged in the crucible of the HIV/AIDS epidemic,[3] when silence, stigma, and indifference cost countless lives. Those of us who lived through that period witnessed how fear supplanted compassion, how patients were left to die alone, and how communities mobilized in defiance. Out of tragedy, activism emerged as both a moral and scientific force. We learned that advancing health equity requires not only evidence but also resistance and, importantly, the education of the health professions workforce.

This conviction has guided our leadership. When I (Halkitis) assumed the role of Dean of the Rutgers School of Public Health, a journalist asked which school I sought to emulate. My response was simple: "None." I wanted to create a model of academic public health that was responsive to the times, reflective of the people it serves, and grounded in the full humanity of those who inhabit it, as well as true to its multidisciplinary ethos.[3]

A modern school of public health must remain expansive, reaching across fields to address the complex forces that shape well-being and embrace a humanized vision of public health.[4] It must be informed by myriad disciplinary perspectives, including but not limited to art, law, medicine, psychology, and urban planning, enabling a biopsychosocial understanding of both disease and well-being.[5–7] That vision led to the creation of the nation's first Master of Public Health concentration in LGBTQ Health at Rutgers, for which I (Krause) served as program director. This program was not designed as an elective curiosity; it was an assertion that LGBTQ health belongs at the center of public health.

Nearly 10% of the US population identifies as lesbian, gay, bisexual, transgender, or queer.[8] Our concentration in LGBTQ public health is as modern and relevant as our other new concentrations in sexual and reproductive health, sustainability and health, population mental health, and population aging—all of which speak to people, their everyday lives, and the support they need to live fuller and healthier lives not only through behavior change but also through understanding of emotions and psychological states, and via activism. Since the concentration's inception, we have expanded our faculty and scholarship, established the first endowed chair in LGBTQ Public Health, launched a Sexual and Gender Minority Health Institute, and founded the *Annals of LGBTQ Public and Population Health*.

These efforts to advance LGBTQ public health have been driven by the persistence of faculty, staff, students, alumni, donors, and allies who refused to accept invisibility. Yet our progress has not come without resistance. We have, more than once, been told by colleagues that "there's too much LGBTQ stuff at the school." Such remarks remind us that for many LGBTQ people in academia, legitimacy remains conditional.

This reality was brought into sharp focus again recently, when a colleague lamented the "lack of male presence" in our student services office—a comment based solely on appearance and

AJPH February 2026, Vol. 116, No. 2

rooted in assumptions about gender identity. Such moments are not merely insensitive; they are injurious. They expose how fragile acceptance can be, even in institutions that publicly champion diversity and inclusion.

The fragility of institutional support mirrors a much broader and more alarming national landscape. In 2025 alone, more than 850 anti-LGBTQ bills were introduced in state legislatures across the country, with dozens enacted into law.[9] These measures curtail access to gender-affirming care, restrict discussions of identity in education, and legitimize discrimination in health care. Earlier this year, federal agencies rescinded dozens of grants supporting LGBTQ health research—only reinstating them after public outrage and legal intervention. Numerous states[10] have put forward measures to restrict new marriage licenses to same-sex couples, and a growing number of public officials and commentators claim there is simply "too much LGBTQ stuff" in American life, as if the mere presence of LGBTQ people and ideas constitutes overreach. Initiatives such as Project 2025[11] explicitly aim to dismantle antidiscrimination protections and erase decades of progress in civil rights.

Yet, when institutions, including academia, falter, LGBTQ people endure. We have always found ways to thrive[12] even when an uncurable infectious disease devastated our communities, emboldening us to innovate to advance the health of our public. Throughout history, our communities have built infrastructures of care in the absence of protection, advancing public health through mutual aid, advocacy, and courage. That same spirit animates the work of our students and graduates today. The LGBTQ Health concentration at Rutgers was not merely added to a curriculum. The program was built from the ground up by those who understood that invisibility is incompatible with equity and who understand that public health is multidisciplinary, and, thus, students learn about social determinants and applied statistical analysis but also LGBTQ history, sampling methods for studies focusing on LGBTQ populations, and communication and humility in working with the populations. This depth in learning advances skills and knowledge in ways that numerous other four- or five-course certificate programs do not.

The "curb-cut effect"[13] offers a powerful metaphor here. Just as curb cuts, designed for wheelchair access, ultimately benefited countless others including parents with strollers, travelers, and delivery workers—so, too, a program like ours strengthens public health as a whole. When we teach cultural humility, trauma-informed care, and gender-affirming approaches, we improve outcomes for all populations. Inclusion is not an accessory to excellence. It is its foundation.

Developing and institutionalizing LGBTQ public health has been one of the most challenging and rewarding undertakings of our careers. It has required perseverance, imagination, and the willingness to challenge old hierarchies. It has also required confronting prejudice—sometimes overt, sometimes subtle—but always real. These encounters hurt, but they also fortify. They remind us that progress in LGBTQ public health, as in all public health, has never been a gift bestowed by institutions. Rather, it has been a fight sustained by people during the Civil Rights Movement who have helped to elevate our nation in incomplete but nonetheless significant ways.

LGBTQ public health is public health. It embodies the field's most noble principles: evidence guided by empathy, science grounded in justice, and policy shaped by humanity. To marginalize it is to misunderstand what public health is meant to be. In this moment—when the rights and health of LGBTQ people are under attack not only by state legislatures but also by the very federal systems and institutions meant to safeguard them[14]—the stakes could not be higher. Too many universities have to make difficult decisions under political and financial pressure to succumb to the current federal administration tactics to silence academic voices and equivocate in the face of LGBTQ hate.[15] More than ever, the responsibility of those of us who lead must be unambiguous. At the Rutgers School of Public Health, and within the broader public health community, we must hold the line. We must continue to teach, to research, to advocate, and to care. Because when institutions falter, we endure—and in doing so, we reaffirm what public health, at its most human, courageous, and just, truly means. AJPH

CORRESPONDENCE

Correspondence should be sent to Perry N. Halkitis, PhD, MS, MPH, One Riverfront Plaza, Suite 1020, Newark, NJ 07102 (e-mail: perry.halkitis@rutgers.edu). Reprints can be ordered at https://www.ajph.org by clicking the "Reprints" link.

PUBLICATION INFORMATION

Full Citation: Halkitis PN, Krause KD. LGBTQ public health is public health: advancing equity when institutions falter. *Am J Public Health*. 2026;116(2): 159–161.

Acceptance Date: November 19, 2025.

DOI: https://doi.org/10.2105/AJPH.2025.308368

ORCID iDs:
Perry N. Halkitis https://orcid.org/0000-0002-1528-4128

Kristen D. Krause https://orcid.org/0000-0001-8761-2314

CONTRIBUTORS

Both authors contributed equally to this work.

CONFLICTS OF INTEREST

The authors have no conflicts of interest to disclose.

REFERENCES

1. Eilola RA. *Barriers and Facilitators to Sexual Orientation Disclosure in Medical Settings: Perspectives From LGBTQ Patients and Healthcare Professionals.* PhD dissertation. Fairfax, Virginia: George Mason University; 2024.
2. McHenry SE. "Gay is good": history of homosexuality in the *DSM* and modern psychiatry. *Am J Psychiatry Resid J.* 2022;18(1):4–5. https://doi.org/10.1176/appi.ajp-rj.2022.180103
3. Halkitis PN. The Stonewall riots, the AIDS epidemic, and the public's health. *Am J Public Health.* 2019;109(6):851–852. https://doi.org/10.2105/AJPH.2019.305079
4. Halkitis PN. *Humanizing Public Health: How Disease-Centered Approaches Have Failed Us.* Baltimore, MD: Johns Hopkins University Press; 2026.
5. Krause KD. Implications of the COVID-19 pandemic on LGBTQ communities. *J Public Health Manag Pract.* 2021;27(suppl 1):S69–S71. https://doi.org/10.1097/PHH.0000000000001273
6. Morris P, Halkitis PN. The influence of context on health. *Behav Med.* 2015;41(3):77–79. https://doi.org/10.1080/08964289.2015.1063869
7. Halkitis PN. A new public health psychology to mend the chasm between public health and clinical care. *Am Psychol.* 2020;75(9):1289–1296. https://doi.org/10.1037/amp0000743
8. Jones JM. LGBTQ+ identification in US rises to 9.3%. *Gallup.* 2025. Available at: https://news.gallup.com/poll/656708/lgbtq-identification-rises.aspx. Accessed December 2, 2025.
9. Reed E. More than 850 anti-LGBTQ bills filed so far in 2025—the most in US history. *Truthout* 2025. Available at: http://truthout.org/articles/more-than-850-anti-lgbtq-bills-filed-so-far-in-2025-the-most-in-us-history. Accessed December 2, 2025.
10. Yurcaba J, Sopelsa B. Lawmakers in 9 states propose measures to undermine same-sex marriage rights. NBC News. 2025. Available at: https://www.nbcnews.com/nbc-out/out-politics-and-policy/lawmakers-9-states-propose-measures-undermine-sex-marriage-rights-rcna193743. Accessed December 2, 2025.
11. ACLU. Project 2025, explained. 2025. Available at: https://www.aclu.org/project-2025-explained. Accessed December 2, 2025.
12. Krause KD, Halkitis PN. Toward a more dynamic understanding of the influence of resilience on health. *Behav Med.* 2020;46(3-4):171–174. https://doi.org/10.1080/08964289.2020.1790972
13. Blackwell AG. The curb-cut effect. *Stanf Soc Innov Rev.* 2016;15(1):28–33.
14. GLAAD. Trump Accountability Tracker. 2025. Available at: https://glaad.org/trump-accountability-tracker. Accessed December 2, 2025.
15. Fulton N. Queer students left holding the line as universities bow to Trump. *Prism.* 2025. Available at: https://prismreports.org/2025/10/02/lgbt-students-colleges-universities. Accessed December 2, 2025.

Short- and Long-Term Potential Impacts of Ongoing and Escalating Legal and Political Attacks on LGBTQ Health and Health Equity

Dougie Zubizarreta, SM, and Ariel L. Beccia, PhD

ABOUT THE AUTHORS

Dougie Zubizarreta is with the Harvard T. H. Chan School of Public Health, Boston, MA. Ariel L. Beccia is with Boston Children's Hospital, Harvard Medical School, and the Harvard T. H. Chan School of Public Health, Boston, MA.

AJPH February 2026, Vol. 116, No. 2

In January 2025, three executive orders were signed—two targeting lesbian, gay, bisexual, transgender, and queer (LGBTQ) populations and one targeting diversity, equity, inclusion, or justice-related efforts—that will affect the present and future of public health and health equity research in unprecedented ways.[1,2] More specifically, Executive Order 14168 seeks to delegitimize gender as a social reality and lived experience and to redefine sex and sex-based discrimination to pertain solely to differences between people assigned male or female at birth, thereby erasing and excluding transgender, nonbinary, and intersex people; 14187 bans the provision of gender-affirming care for transgender people younger than 19 years; and 14151 terminates all programs, policies, and other initiatives pertaining to diversity, equity, inclusion, or justice.

We posit that these executive orders, regardless of their legal status, are manifestations of structural cisheterosexism, a root cause of LGBTQ-related health inequities that encompasses laws and policies, institutionalized practices, and cultural norms that systematically restrict access to power, resources, and opportunities for LGBTQ people while privileging their cisgender and heterosexual peers.[3] Structural forms of discrimination, including structural cisheterosexism, influence inequitable distributions of social determinants of health, including educational and economic resources and opportunities, resulting in individual-level harms to LGBTQ people and population-level LGBTQ-related health inequities.[3] These and other related executive orders (e.g., 14173 targets diversity-, equity-, and inclusion-related initiatives; 14190 eliminates federal funding for K–12 schools that promote "gender ideology"; 14201 bans transgender women from sports; and 14183 bans transgender people from military service) have already had devastating effects on the health and well-being of LGBTQ people broadly, including LGBTQ scientists.[1,4,5]

For example, several immediate impacts include elimination of federal funding for LGBTQ-related health services (including HIV prevention and treatment), restriction of access to gender-affirming care for transgender youths, censoring of sexual orientation and gender identity data from public health surveillance systems, and termination of federally funded LGBTQ-related grants.[1,4,5] Moreover, these executive orders and broader related political ideologies and agendas will likely have long-term impacts on public health and health equity research unless we take immediate action.[1,6]

POSITIONALITY

In December 2024, we each began preparing National Institutes of Health (NIH) grants. Ariel L. Beccia, as a postdoctoral fellow at Harvard Medical School with previous NIH F32 (postdoctoral fellowship) and F31 (predoctoral fellowship) funding, applied for a K01 award (mentored career development award). Dougie Zubizarreta, as a doctoral student at the Harvard T. H. Chan School of Public Health, applied for an F31 award. As queer junior scholars focused on structural drivers of LGBTQ-related health inequities, navigating the NIH grant process in the post-inauguration sociopolitical climate was incredibly stressful.

For example, given that her F32 fellowship was abruptly terminated in the slew of attacks on NIH grants, would Beccia have a salary and health insurance coverage if her K01 award was not funded because of its focus on LGBTQ health? Would the data sources we each planned to use (and currently use in our day-to-day work)—which include national health surveillance systems, large-scale NIH cohorts, and foundational population data from the US Census Bureau—remain publicly available, and, if not, would they be retrievable through web archives?

We were also anxious about the future. For example, would postdoctoral fellowships and faculty positions still exist for researchers who specialize in LGBTQ health, health equity, or structural discrimination research, and would we be able to secure funding to cover our salaries? What about the careers of our colleagues and mentors and the dedicated LGBTQ resources, programs, and centers that have only recently been increasingly founded and funded? As junior researchers, we feared being viewed as more expendable, and thus experiencing greater occupational precarity, given our relatively limited experience in the field. More broadly, we feared the short- and long-term impacts of these legal and political attacks on LGBTQ health research and the potential implications with respect to the loss of dedicated services, resources, and information to protect and improve the health and well-being of LGBTQ people.

Furthermore, these executive orders are simultaneously affecting both the professional work and personal lives of many LGBTQ health researchers. For example, transgender scholars conducting transgender health research not only confront the decimation of their field but also face severe restrictions of their rights to legally and medically transition. International LGBTQ health researchers—many of whom came to the United States because it has historically provided opportunities to conduct LGBTQ health research—now face legal threats jeopardizing their ability to complete their degree programs. These examples highlight how these executive orders may disproportionately affect people whose lived experiences are shaped by the compounding adverse impacts of intersecting systems of power and oppression.

IMPLICATIONS FOR CAREER DEVELOPMENT OPPORTUNITIES

The aforementioned executive orders and the corresponding attacks on LGBTQ health research and researchers have significant implications for career development, particularly with respect to funding, training, and employment opportunities. Between February 28 and April 28, 2025, an estimated 524 NIH grants were terminated because of their focus, to varying extents, on LGBTQ health.[7] Consequently, many junior scholars have been affected; specifically, it is estimated that 47 of these grants were training-focused grants (F31, F32, R36) awarded to doctoral students and postdoctoral fellows, 16 were career development–focused grants (K01, K99/R00) awarded to early-career scholars, and 23 were grants supporting institutional training programs providing research training opportunities to doctoral students and postdoctoral fellows (T32).

Also of note, the NIH has terminated the F31 diversity mechanism, which was designed to support doctoral trainees from underrepresented backgrounds (e.g., those with a disability or those who are from a socioeconomically disadvantaged background) in receiving highly specialized training while leading research as principal investigators. The termination of this mechanism, which occurred regardless of the scientific premise of the funded grants, ultimately targeted researchers' identities that the government previously classified as eligibility criteria for the award.[8]

Importantly, the aforementioned training- and career development–focused grants typically cover salary, health insurance, and work-related travel for junior researchers. The harms that these cuts will cause cannot be overstated. As is true for much of science, public health research broadly and health equity research specifically are largely funded through NIH grants. Alternative funding sources include foundation grants or philanthropy; notably, however, such sources are relatively small relative to NIH grants (e.g., \$1000–\$10 000 vs \$40 000–\$90 000) and are typically limited in duration and allowable expenses (e.g., most do not allow for salary to be covered, and expenses are often restricted to data access and collection, open-access publication fees, and software and equipment). As a result, in only a couple of months, the field of LGBTQ health research has been decimated.

Moreover, junior researchers whose own grants were terminated—as well as those whose mentors' grants were terminated—are at immediate risk for losing their salary, benefits, health insurance, and potentially even employment. More broadly, given the looming threats of continued grant terminations and other federal funding cuts, a growing number of higher education institutions across the United States have implemented hiring freezes, restricting employment opportunities for junior researchers at critical junctures in their career development (e.g., transitions from doctoral student to postdoctoral fellow and from postdoctoral fellow to tenure-track positions).[9]

IMPLICATIONS FOR RESEARCH: PRESENT AND FUTURE

Termination of NIH-funded grants related to LGBTQ health and health equity–related topics has coincided with governmental efforts to limit and, in some cases, ban efforts to monitor the health and well-being of LGBTQ populations through public health surveillance systems.[6] After the inauguration, the NIH disbanded the Sexual & Gender Minority Research Office,[10] which was specifically dedicated to advancing health equity for LGBTQ populations and coordinated all relevant research efforts within the agency, including creating and disseminating resources on best practices in sexual orientation and gender identity measurement for health research.[11] Then, on February 25, 2025, the Centers for Disease Control and Prevention announced that it would stop processing "transgender data," meaning that our largest public health surveillance systems (e.g., the Behavioral Risk Factor Surveillance System, the Youth Risk Behavior Surveillance System) will no longer collect or analyze gender identity data, precluding documentation and thus action to address LGBTQ-related health inequities at the state and national levels.[6,12]

Banning efforts to collect information on gender identity—and potentially sexual orientation—by any institution receiving federal funding over the next four years will create immeasurable knowledge gaps regarding the health and well-being of LGBTQ populations. Of note, an estimated one in five youths born between 1997 and 2012 ("Generation Z") and nearly one in 10 adults aged 18 years or older identify as LGBTQ.[13] Also, as noted, LGBTQ populations face pronounced, persistent, and pervasive physical and mental health inequities, with even greater inequities documented among multiply marginalized populations.[14] Previous research has shown that increases in structural discrimination, including passing or even introducing[15] discriminatory laws and policies, are linked to increases in adverse health outcomes and widening inequities for LGBTQ people.[14] Given the ongoing and escalating attacks on LGBTQ populations' rights, health, and well-being, the lack of data tracking the health of these populations will directly hinder efforts to resist structural discrimination and advance equity.

CENSORSHIP AND IMPLICATIONS FOR HEALTH EQUITY

The recent executive orders and corresponding circulating lists of "banned words" (Box 1) have introduced a chilling effect on science.[16] While developing our NIH grants, we were forced to confront the difficult decision of whether and, if so, how to modify our applications to comply (e.g., which language to use or avoid, which sections to censor or leave uncensored), a shared experience among health equity researchers currently applying for federal funding.[17] Ultimately, we decided to remove any "banned words" from our public-facing materials (i.e., the title, project narrative, and project summary/abstract). We also attempted to broaden the focus of our proposals to make them applicable to several NIH agencies rather than pigeonholed into one, given looming threats of restructuring and cuts.

The extent to which such censorship will influence the conduct of research on LGBTQ health and health equity moving forward is unknown. That said, it means that fellow researchers, when searching NIH Reporter for similar grants, will likely face challenges in understanding what previous studies have focused on, reducing both transparency and the ability to build on one another's work.

FUTURE DIRECTIONS AND OPPORTUNITIES TO TAKE ACTION

Although lawsuits are under way to resist the attacks on LGBTQ health and health equity research,[18] researchers and particularly junior researchers are in need of immediate support. Academic institutions are uniquely positioned to take action to protect and promote the careers of LGBTQ health and health equity researchers. First and foremost, institutions should bridge affected researchers' salaries through alternative

BOX 1— Select List of Banned or Flagged Words and Phrases to Be Avoided by Federal Agencies According to a Compilation of Government Documents: January 21, 2025, to Present

LGBTQ-Specific Terms	Health Equity–Relevant Terms
Assigned male/female at birth	Advocacy
Female (but not male)	Antiracist
Gender identity	Barriers
Gender-affirming care	DEI
LGBTQ	Disparity
Men who have sex with men	Equity
Nonbinary	Inequity
Pronouns	Intersectionality
Sexual preference	Marginalized
Transgender	Oppression
Women (but not men)	Vulnerable populations

Note. DEI = diversity, equity, and inclusion; LGBTQ = lesbian, gay, bisexual, transgender, and queer.

funding streams (e.g., hard money from teaching or committee service), particularly for those whose grants were unjustly and prematurely terminated. Relatedly, they can offer dedicated internal grant opportunities or emergency continuity funds alongside removing indirect cost requirements that often preclude researchers from applying for smaller foundation grants that may be especially well suited for health equity work.

Beyond funding, institutions can support (junior) LGBTQ health researchers in myriad ways, including termination appeal guidance if or when relevant, legal and mental health resources, enhanced mentorship, tenure clock extensions, and public statements affirming their commitment to researchers' lines of work. In addition, we recommend that early-career researchers consider expanding their professional networks and affiliations beyond academic institutions—such as by establishing clinical partnerships and seeking appointments at research or policy institutes—and then leverage these nonacademic affiliations and collaborations to apply for funding opportunities to help ensure research and funding continuity.

Moreover, it is critical to support LGBTQ health researchers in pursuing scientific communication and public engagement opportunities (e.g., media interviews, community events) to help inform the public about how these executive orders will adversely affect LGBTQ health and health equity in the United States. Such outreach has been and will continue to be essential for raising awareness, combating misinformation, and garnering broader support in resistance efforts. Across the board, there is an urgent need for dedicated support, both material and moral, of LGBTQ health research and researchers by the academic community. This represents one way in which we can collectively start to address the escalating cisheterosexist attacks and advance equity. AJPH

CORRESPONDENCE

Correspondence should be sent to Dougie Zubizarreta, SM, Department of Social and Behavioral Sciences, Harvard T. H. Chan School of Public Health, 677 Huntington Ave, Boston, MA 02115 (e-mail: dzubizarreta@hsph.harvard.edu). Reprints can be ordered at https://www.ajph.org by clicking the "Reprints" link.

PUBLICATION INFORMATION

Full Citation: Zubizarreta D, Beccia AL. Short- and long-term potential impacts of ongoing and escalating legal and political attacks on LGBTQ health and health equity. *Am J Public Health*. 2026;116(2): 162–165.

Acceptance Date: July 29, 2025.

DOI: https://doi.org/10.2105/AJPH.2025.308261

ORCID iD:
Dougie Zubizarreta https://orcid.org/0000-0003-2098-6404

CONTRIBUTORS

Both authors contributed to conceptualization and the writing of the original draft.

CONFLICTS OF INTEREST

The authors have no conflicts of interest to disclose.

REFERENCES

1. Medina C, Babbs G, Mar S, Hughto JMW, Tobin-Tyler E. What do the Trump executive orders mean for the health of trans Americans? *Health Affairs*. Available at: https://www.healthaffairs.org/content/forefront/do-trump-executive-orders-mean-health-trans-americans. Accessed April 14, 2025.
2. Executive Office of the President. Ending radical and wasteful government DEI programs and preferencing. Available at: https://www.federalregister.gov/documents/2025/01/29/2025-01953/ending-radical-and-wasteful-government-dei-programs-and-preferencing. Accessed April 14, 2025.
3. Krieger N. Measures of racism, sexism, heterosexism, and gender binarism for health equity research: from structural injustice to embodied harm—an ecosocial analysis. *Annu Rev Public Health*. 2020;41:37–62. https://doi.org/10.1146/annurev-publhealth-040119-094017
4. LGBTQ+ Bar. Trump anti-LGBTQ+ executive order litigation tracker. Available at: https://lgbtqbar.org/programs/trump-executive-order-tracker. Accessed June 28, 2025.
5. Dawson L, Kates J. Overview of President Trump's executive actions impacting LGBTQ+ health. KFF. Available at: https://www.kff.org/other/fact-sheet/overview-of-president-trumps-executive-actions-impacting-lgbtq-health. Accessed June 28, 2025.
6. The Codcast. The data purge domino effect. Available at: https://commonwealthbeacon.org/the-codcast/the-data-purge-domino-effect. Accessed June 28, 2025.
7. Airtable. NIH grant terminations in 2025. Available at: https://airtable.com/appjhyo9NTvJLocRy/shrNto1NNp9eJlgpA?Ffj6Q%3Asort=eyJwZWwxbIJuTkNGdW9YWDNjRiI6eyJjb2x1bW5JZCI6ImZsZGlIUG1FU3NCTDZEMnRlIiwiYXNjZW5kaW5nIjp0cnVlfX0&Ffj6Q=sfsHYOnE89ibBCJBT. Accessed March 29, 2025.
8. National Institutes of Health. Rescinded: Notice of Civil Rights Term and Condition of Award. Available at: https://grants.nih.gov/grants/guide/notice-files/NOT-OD-25-090.html. Accessed June 28, 2025.
9. Treisman R. Universities across the US freeze hiring as federal funding hangs in the balance. National Public Radio. Available at: https://www.npr.org/2025/03/12/nx-s1-5324496/universities-hiring-freezes-federal-funding. Accessed March 29, 2025.
10. Gaffney T. NIH puts former Sexual & Gender Minority Office employees on administrative leave. *STAT News*. Available at: https://www.statnews.com/2025/03/06/nih-puts-former-sexual-and-gender-minority-office-employees-on-administrative-leave. Accessed March 29, 2025.
11. National Institutes of Health. Methods and measurement in sexual and gender minority health: developing a research agenda and identifying research opportunities. Available at: https://web.archive.org/web/20240327062641/https://dpcpsi.nih.gov/sites/default/files/MethodsMeasures_Paper_508_FV.pdf. Accessed April 4, 2025.
12. Gaffney T. CDC will no longer process transgender data. *STAT News*. Available at: https://www.statnews.com/2025/02/25/cdc-will-no-longer-process-transgender-data. Accessed April 4, 2025.
13. Jones JM. LGBTQ+ identification in US now at 7.6%. Gallup. Available at: https://news.gallup.com/poll/611864/lgbtq-identification.aspx. Accessed May 29, 2025.
14. Hatzenbuehler ML, Lattanner MR, McKetta S, Pachankis JE. Structural stigma and LGBTQ+ health: a narrative review of quantitative studies. *Lancet Public Health*. 2024;9(2):e109–e127. https://doi.org/10.1016/S2468-2667(23)00312-2
15. Horne SG, McGinley M, Yel N, Maroney MR. The stench of bathroom bills and anti-transgender legislation: anxiety and depression among transgender, nonbinary, and cisgender LGBQ people during a state referendum. *J Couns Psychol*. 2022;69(1):1–13. https://doi.org/10.1037/cou0000558
16. Yourish K, Daniel A, Datar S, White I, Gamio L. These words are disappearing in the new Trump administration. *NY Times*. Available at: https://www.nytimes.com/interactive/2025/03/07/us/trump-federal-agencies-websites-words-dei.html. Accessed April 4, 2025.
17. Lee McFarling U, Chen A, Owermohle S. Growing number of federal health agencies are combing grants for taboo words, unnerving researchers. *STAT News*. Available at: https://www.statnews.com/2025/02/13/trump-dei-ban-banned-words-list-scrambles-research-nih-veterans-affairs/#:~:text=It%20included%20%E2%80%9Cbiased%2C%E2%80%9D%20%E2%80%9C,or%20the%20microbiome%20or%20galaxies. Accessed March 29, 2025.
18. Jones N. NIH cuts triggered a host of lawsuits: *Nature*'s guide to what's next. *Nature*. Available at: https://www.nature.com/articles/d41586-025-01192-y. Accessed May 2, 2025.

The Urgent Need for Evidence and Action on Global Transgender Mental Health

Ayden I. Scheim, PhD

ABOUT THE AUTHOR

Ayden I. Scheim is with the Williams Institute, School of Law, University of California, Los Angeles, and the Department of Epidemiology and Biostatistics, Schulich School of Medicine and Dentistry, Western University, London, ON.

See also Coelho et al., p. 261.

AJPH February 2026, Vol. 116, No. 2

Globally, transgender, nonbinary, and other gender-diverse ("trans") people are facing coordinated and unrelenting attacks on their dignity, health, safety, and civil rights. Against this backdrop, the lived realities of trans communities are highly heterogeneous, and in many parts of the world, these attacks are far from new. Although anti-transgender rhetoric reached a crescendo under former president Jair Bolsonaro, Brazil has long stood out as the country with the largest number of recorded murders of trans people (https://bit.ly/4rdjEtb). It is important to note that these data also reflect the organizing and recordkeeping capacity of trans movements in the absence of inclusion in official statistics. In this context, it is vital to identify and address the wide-ranging health consequences of structural and interpersonal stigma and violence trans people experience worldwide.

Minority stress models situate mental health disparities affecting trans populations as resulting from exposure to distal (e.g., discrimination) and proximal (e.g., internalized stigma) stressors tied to minoritized social identities and positions.[1,2] Numerous studies, largely from the United States, have demonstrated that minority stressors contribute to the high burden of suicidality among trans people.[3] In the Global South, however, research on trans health has focused primarily on HIV, which does not reflect the expressed health priorities of trans communities.[4]

In this issue of *AJPH*, Coehlo et al. (p. 261) report baseline data from an ongoing cohort study of transgender women and *travestis* in Rio de Janeiro, Brazil. (*Travesti* is a transfeminine identity specific to Latin America, particularly Brazil, and often serving as a political identity denoting social marginalization.) About half of participants reported lifetime suicidality, and among those with suicidal ideation, more than half had attempted suicide. Notably, the burden of suicidality did not decrease over the study period (2015–2023). Consistent with the gender minority stress framework, the authors found that lifetime discrimination based on gender identity and experiences of sexual assault were associated with increased suicidality, whereas higher body satisfaction was associated with lower suicidality.

Older age, good self-rated health, and self-reports of living with HIV were also associated with lower odds of suicidality in multivariable analyses. The last finding was unexpected but may reflect the inclusion of participants from a clinical cohort of people with HIV. In many settings, people with diagnosed HIV who are engaged in care have access to dedicated, holistic health and social services. These programs address health and social needs that trans people commonly experience, underscoring the importance of offering status-neutral services that serve trans people regardless of HIV status; such services may also reduce HIV stigma.

Coehlo et al. drew on suicide ideation-to-action frameworks to analyze suicidality as an ordinal outcome that progresses from no suicidality to suicidal ideation and ultimately to both ideation and attempts. These frameworks emphasize the need to identify factors distinguishing those who attempt suicide from those who experience only ideation.[3] To inform suicide prevention interventions—particularly given the very high prevalence of suicide ideation among trans people in this study and globally—future research could focus on predictors of attempts among those with ideation. For example, previous research in Canada identified an elevated risk of suicide attempts (but not ideation) among those in the process of medical gender transition; this has critical implications for prevention strategies.[5] Using longitudinal data or past-year measures to identify factors associated with recent suicidality would also help to inform interventions. Research is urgently needed to identify modifiable factors linked specifically to recent suicide attempts.

This does not imply that there should be a sole focus on individual-level interventions. Stigma and discrimination are modifiable, as are health policies that restrict access to gender-affirming care. As Coehlo et al. suggest, legal protections for trans people, enforcement of existing protections, and expansion of publicly funded gender-affirming care are critical strategies for mitigating mental health inequities. Yet in the face of worsening social and political conditions for trans people, immediate and proximal interventions are also needed. In addition to strengthening formal health and social services, interventions can build on and financially support existing trans community strengths. Trans communities have long organized to provide mutual support—including health care, housing, and self-defense training—that can reduce exposure to violence, buffer the effects of discrimination, and promote protective factors such as body satisfaction.

Coehlo et al. should be commended for using the robust infrastructure of their HIV-focused cohort to address other pressing health issues among *travestis* and trans women in Brazil. A narrow emphasis on HIV neglects health issues of high priority to trans communities and may paradoxically alienate trans people from HIV-related research and services.

Also urgent is addressing the historic exclusion of transmasculine people from global trans health research, despite evidence of similar mental health needs. A recent scoping review of 46 Brazilian trans health studies found only three that reported disaggregated quantitative data on transmasculine persons,[6] reflecting a global research gap.[7] Two of these studies found similar levels of mental distress among transmasculine compared with transfeminine participants,[8,9] underscoring the need for gender-inclusive research. At the same time, considering the distinct social positions and experiences of transmasculine people, gender-specific research is also warranted.[10] Recent participatory surveys of transmasculine communities in Argentina[11] and India[12] revealed high levels of mental health distress and health care barriers, highlighting both the feasibility and the urgency of such research. To maximize the relevance and impact of trans health research, it is imperative that researchers draw on the expertise and insight of trans community members. Community-based participatory approaches, ideally those engaging trans people as equal partners in shaping research, offer a model for ensuring that research agendas and outcomes align with community priorities. AJPH

CORRESPONDENCE

Correspondence should be sent to Ayden I. Scheim, The Williams Institute, UCLA School of Law, 385 Charles E Young Dr E, Los Angeles, CA 90095 (e-mail: drascheim@gmail.com). Reprints can be ordered at https://www.ajph.org by clicking the "Reprints" link.

PUBLICATION INFORMATION

Full Citation: Scheim AI. The urgent need for evidence and action on global transgender mental health. *Am J Public Health*. 2026;116(2):166–167.

Acceptance Date: November 9, 2025.

DOI: https://doi.org/10.2105/AJPH.2025.308356

ORCID iD:
Ayden I. Scheim https://orcid.org/0000-0001-8498-9829

CONFLICTS OF INTEREST

The author has no conflicts of interest to disclose.

REFERENCES

1. Brooks VR. *Minority Stress and Lesbian Women*. Lanham, MD: Lexington Books; 1981.
2. Hendricks ML, Testa RJ. A conceptual framework for clinical work with transgender and gender nonconforming clients: an adaptation of the minority stress model. *Prof Psychol Res Pr*. 2012; 43(5):460–467. https://doi.org/10.1037/a0029597
3. Wolford-Clevenger C, Frantell K, Smith PN, Flores LY, Stuart GL. Correlates of suicide ideation and behaviors among transgender people: a systematic review guided by ideation-to-action theory. *Clin Psychol Rev*. 2018;63:93–105. https://doi.org/10.1016/j.cpr.2018.06.009
4. Thomas R, Pega F, Khosla R, Verster A, Hana T, Say L. Ensuring an inclusive global health agenda for transgender people. *Bull World Health Organ*. 2017;95(2):154–156. https://doi.org/10.2471/BLT.16.183913
5. Bauer GR, Scheim AI, Pyne J, Travers R, Hammond R. Intervenable factors associated with suicide risk in transgender persons: a respondent-driven sampling study in Ontario, Canada. *BMC Public Health*. 2015;15:525. https://doi.org/10.1186/s12889-015-1867-2
6. Freitas FLS, Bermudez X, Merchan-Hamann E, Dias Dos Santos AS, Vieira VF. Social and programmatic vulnerability in the context of transgender people's health: a scoping review of scientific evidence from Brazil. *Int J Equity Health*. 2024;23(1):272. https://doi.org/10.1186/s12939-024-02359-1
7. Scheim A, Kacholia V, Logie C, Chakrapani V, Ranade K, Gupta S. Health of transgender men in low-income and middle-income countries: a scoping review. *BMJ Glob Health*. 2020;5(11): e003471. https://doi.org/10.1136/bmjgh-2020-003471
8. Corrêa FHM, Rodrigues BB, Mendonça JC, Cruz L. Pensamento suicida entre a população transgênero: um estudo epidemiológico [Suicidal thoughts among a transgender population: an epidemiological study]. *J Bras Psiquiatr*. 2020; 69(1):13–22. https://doi.org/10.1590/0047-2085000000256
9. Lobato MI, Soll BM, Costa AB, et al. Psychological distress among transgender people in Brazil: frequency, intensity and social causation—an *ICD-11* field study. *Braz J Psychiatry*. 2019;41(4): 310–315. https://doi.org/10.1590/1516-4446-2018-0052
10. Restar A, Jin H, Operario D. Gender-inclusive and gender-specific approaches in trans health research. *Transgend Health*. 2021;6(5):235–239. https://doi.org/10.1089/trgh.2020.0054
11. Caballero R, Radusky PD, Zalazar V, et al. Psychosocial factors associated with non-suicidal self-injury attempts among people in the transmasculine and non-binary spectrum from Argentina. *Psychol Sex*. 2024;16(1):86–97.
12. Chakrapani V, Santos H, Battala M, et al. Access to transition-related health care among transmasculine people in India: a mixed-methods investigation. *PLoS Glob Public Health*. 2024;4(10): e0003506. https://doi.org/10.1371/journal.pgph.0003506

How Political Dynamics May Shape Availability and Utilization of Health Care Services Through Federally Qualified Health Centers

Eun Kyung Lee, PhD, MPH, and Megan B. Cole, PhD, MPH

ABOUT THE AUTHORS

Eun Kyung Lee is with the Department of Environmental Studies, SUNY College of Environmental Science and Forestry, Syracuse, NY. Megan B. Cole is with the Department of Population Medicine, Harvard Medical School and Harvard Pilgrim Health Care Institute, Boston, MA.

See also Côté-L'Heureux and Chin, p. 270.

Previous research indicates that civic engagement and political advocacy are associated with improved health outcomes.[1] Yet, political representation remains uneven, and organizations such as federally qualified health centers (FQHCs)—which rely heavily on public funding through federal grants, Medicaid dollars, and local investment—are particularly vulnerable to political influence. These dynamics shape both the social and physical environments in which people live, perpetuating health disparities and unmet health and social needs. Such pressures increasingly threaten the sustainability of FQHCs. However, little is known about how divisions in political representation—particularly those driven by gerrymandering (i.e., the manipulation of electoral district boundaries to benefit particular political, racial, or socioeconomic groups) and racial segregation—affect FQHC availability.

HOW POLITICAL BOUNDARIES SHAPE HEALTH CARE ACCESS

Côté-L'Heureux and Chin examined the relationship between gerrymandering and the distribution of FQHCs in North Carolina (p. 270). Using publicly available precinct-level voter registration data and FQHC information from the Health Resources and Services Administration's (HRSA's) Uniform Data System (2004–2022), they developed novel metrics to quantify local gerrymandering. These metrics captured both "voter dislocation" and "uncertainty of district membership," accounting both for political party and racial splits within each measure.

FQHCs are federally funded, community-based health care facilities that primarily serve marginalized populations. Their mission is to deliver comprehensive, culturally competent, high-quality primary care without regard for ability to pay.[2] Historically, FQHCs have been instrumental in expanding and facilitating access to health care and have grown exponentially in recent years. In 2024, FQHCs served approximately 34 million individuals, roughly one in 10 people in the United States. Among those served, nearly 90% were below 200% of the federal poverty level, 64% were publicly insured, 18% were uninsured, and 64% identified as members of racial or ethnic minority groups.[3]

Federal regulations partly dictate where FQHCs can be located, restricting their placement to either (1) medically underserved areas—regions with limited access to primary care[4] or (2) areas serving medically underserved populations, where specific groups of people experience cultural, linguistic, or insurance-related barriers to care. However, the availability of FQHC services is increasingly threatened. One imminent threat includes reductions in insurance coverage and Medicaid funding, because of recent policy changes and federal funding cuts resulting from the One Big Beautiful Bill Act of 2025. The sustainment of FQHC services is also threatened by longstanding systemic underinvestment in historically marginalized communities.

While FQHCs help address unmet social needs—for example, by providing transportation to appointments, care coordination, and assistance with safety-net enrollment—the growing prevalence of these needs, driven by persistent local underinvestment, may hinder their ability to sustain comprehensive support. These fiscal and structural pressures may precipitate staff reductions or site closures, or limit new site development, particularly in communities with the greatest need.

During large-scale crises such as the COVID-19 pandemic, these vulnerabilities become particularly consequential, as underserved populations experience disproportionate health and social burdens.[5] As emphasized by Côté-L'Heureux and Chin, political forces and power dynamics have emerged as critical, yet underexamined factors influencing the geographic distribution and sustainability of FQHCs.

The authors identified several key findings. First, gerrymandering was inversely associated with the availability of and access to FQHCs across North Carolina. Both partisan and racial gerrymandering showed significant negative associations with FQHC availability and utilization, particularly at the state legislative district and congressional district levels. Communities that were split across district boundaries were significantly less likely to gain new FQHCs over time. Second, in urban areas, state legislative district–level partisan and racial gerrymandering had the strongest negative impact on both FQHC availability and patient volume. In rural areas, less gerrymandering was significantly associated with increased FQHC availability, although congressional district–level dislocation still increased distance to care at FQHCs. Third, higher electoral entropy (i.e., more competitive or fragmented elections) was linked to lower FQHC availability and patient volume. Meanwhile, residential segregation by race or political party was correlated with voter dislocation but not directly with FQHC access. These findings suggest that structural political factors may exacerbate existing inequities in health care access.

Their findings highlight the importance of addressing health care access shortages by considering political and policy determinants that shape service availability, complementing previous research on how residential segregation undermines health care access for vulnerable populations.[6,7] Previous research indicates that FQHCs can mitigate disparities in access to health care, particularly in historically redlined neighborhoods, underscoring their disproportionate role in addressing structural inequities.[8] While FQHC access has expanded nationwide, especially in lower income and higher-vulnerability areas, the increase of gerrymandering and resulting splits in political representation may threaten this progress. These patterns emphasize the need to examine political forces shaping access to essential health services—forces that may jeopardize the advances achieved through FQHC expansion.

THE PRESENT AND FUTURE EFFECTS OF US GERRYMANDERING

The ongoing national debate over gerrymandering in states such as Texas and California underscores the urgency of understanding how political dynamics, especially manipulative practices that may shift electoral outcomes, impact health care. As the two most populous and demographically diverse states—together home to more than 70 million Americans—Texas and California present a compelling context for examining how electoral boundaries and political power structures impact the distribution of health care resources. In Texas, for instance, significant barriers to care persist: 18.6% of residents remain uninsured, and 17.4% of adults report not seeing a doctor in the past year—the highest rates in the nation.[9,10] Recent approvals of gerrymandered district maps in both states are projected to flip several congressional seats, potentially exacerbating existing barriers to health care.

Several mechanisms may explain the ill effects of gerrymandering on health care access—including FQHC access—in Texas, California, and elsewhere. First, as described by Côté-L'Heureux and Chin, gerrymandering may split communities in a way that results in less civic and community engagement. Because FQHC boards must be governed by at least 51% patient representation from the community, lesser engagement within the community may result in a lesser likelihood of opening a new FQHC site or may threaten the longer-term sustainability of existing FQHCs if community engagement declines.

Second, FQHC operations also depend on stable revenue streams. The two main sources of FQHC revenue are (1) federal grants from the HRSA, which are determined by federally established formulas but require broader, politically influenced Congressional action, and (2) Medicaid patient revenue, where total FQHC Medicaid revenue is closely linked to state Medicaid policies such as Medicaid eligibility expansions, which are highly political.

Finally, FQHC access reflects broader state and local policy priorities. Political parties that underinvest in health care, education, and social services contribute to rising unmet social needs in their constituencies. Addressing both the health and social needs of patients, including direct provision of social supports, is core to the FQHC mission; yet, as community needs rise without corresponding increases in federal funding, the ability of FQHCs to sustain services is increasingly threatened.

Ultimately, understanding the political and funding mechanisms that influence availability and utilization of health services—especially at FQHCs—is urgent, as these factors may directly shape disparities in disease burden, reliance on emergency departments, and, in extreme cases, mortality.[11] Looking ahead, measuring and improving civic engagement as a determinant of health is increasingly important. Initiatives such as Vot-ER, which embed nonpartisan voter registration into clinical workflows, illustrate how civic participation can be mobilized within health care settings.[12] More broadly, civic engagement and voting should be recognized as critical social determinants of health, as they enhance the political and social capital of marginalized populations, empower communities to advocate for essential needs, and promote equitable, community-responsive access to health care. As gerrymandering efforts persist across states, mitigating its impacts on civic engagement and, ultimately, health care access is essential; otherwise, health inequities will continue to grow. AJPH

CORRESPONDENCE

Correspondence should be sent to Eun Kyung Lee, One Forestry Drive, Syracuse, NY 13210 (e-mail: eklee02@esf.edu). Reprints can be ordered at https://www.ajph.org by clicking the "Reprints" link.

PUBLICATION INFORMATION

Full Citation: Lee EK, Cole MB. How political dynamics may shape availability and utilization of health care services through federally qualified health centers. *Am J Public Health*. 2026;116(2): 168–170.

Acceptance Date: November 17, 2025.

DOI: https://doi.org/10.2105/AJPH.2025.308367

ORCID iDs:

Eun Kyung Lee https://orcid.org/0000-0002-9917-0928

Megan B. Cole https://orcid.org/0000-0001-8731-4210

CONTRIBUTORS

Both authors provided substantial contributions to the conceptualization and interpretation of the editorial, contributed substantially to drafting the work and revising it critically for important intellectual content, provided the final approval of the version to be published, and agree to be accountable for all aspects of the work in ensuring that questions related to the accuracy or integrity of any part of the work are appropriately investigated and resolved.

ACKNOWLEDGMENTS

The authors would like to thank the editors and anonymous reviewers for their thoughtful and timely reviews, which improved the quality of this editorial.

CONFLICTS OF INTEREST

The authors report no conflicts of interest.

REFERENCES

1. Dubowitz T, Nelson C, Weilant S, et al. Factors related to health civic engagement: results from the 2018 National Survey of Health Attitudes to understand progress towards a Culture of Health. *BMC Public Health*. 2020;20(1):635. https://doi.org/10.1186/s12889-020-08507-w
2. Health Resources and Services Administration. What is a health center? 2016. Available at: https://bphc.hrsa.gov/about/what-is-a-health-center/index.html. Accessed May 16, 2022.
3. Health Resources and Services Administration. Impact of the health center program. August 2025. Available at: https://bphc.hrsa.gov/about-health-center-program/impact-health-center-program. Accessed September 8, 2025.
4. Health Resources and Services Administration. Find MUA/P. 2022. Available at: https://data.hrsa.gov/tools/shortage-area/mua-find. Accessed April 24, 2022.
5. Cole MB, Lee EK, Frogner BK, Wright B. Changes in performance measures and service volume at US federally qualified health centers during the COVID-19 pandemic. *JAMA Health Forum*. 2023;4(4):e230351. https://doi.org/10.1001/jamahealthforum.2023.0351
6. Ko M, Ponce NA. Community residential segregation and the local supply of federally qualified health centers. *Health Serv Res*. 2013;48(1): 253–270. https://doi.org/10.1111/j.1475-6773.2012.01444.x
7. Gaskin DJ, Dinwiddie GY, Chan KS, McCleary R. Residential segregation and disparities in health care services utilization. *Med Care Res Rev*. 2012;69(2):158–175. https://doi.org/10.1177/1077558711420263
8. Lee EK, Donley G, Ciesielski TH, Freedman DA, Cole MB. Spatial availability of federally qualified health centers and disparities in health services utilization in medically underserved areas. *Soc Sci Med*. 2023;328:116009. https://doi.org/10.1016/j.socscimed.2023.116009
9. Tolbert J, Cervantes S, Bell C, Damico A. Key facts about the uninsured population. KFF. December 18, 2024. Available at: https://www.kff.org/uninsured/key-facts-about-the-uninsured-population. Accessed October 2, 2025.
10. Kaiser Family Foundation. Adults who report not seeing a doctor in the past 12 months because of cost by sex. 2024. Available at: https://www.kff.org/state-health-policy-data/state-indicator/could-not-see-doctor-because-of-cost-by-sex/?currentTimeframe=0&sortModel=%7B%22colId%22:%22Location%22,%22sort%22:%22asc%22%7D. Accessed October 2, 2025.
11. Myong C, Hull P, Price M, Hsu J, Newhouse JP, Fung V. The impact of funding for federally qualified health centers on utilization and emergency department visits in Massachusetts. *PLoS One*. 2020;15(12):e0243279. https://doi.org/10.1371/journal.pone.0243279
12. Martin A, Betancourt J. Beyond the exam room: impacting health outcomes through civic engagement. Grants Makers in Health. August 15, 2025. Available at: https://www.gih.org/views-from-the-field/beyond-the-exam-room-impacting-health-outcomes-through-civic-engagement. Accessed September 8, 2025.

Disaster Within a Disaster: Ensuring Access to Opioid Use Disorder Treatment During Natural Crises

Elizabeth Cerceo, MD, DCM, Cordelia Stearns, MD, Kathleen Shapley-Quinn, MD, DCM, and Matthew Salzman, MD

ABOUT THE AUTHORS

Elizabeth Cerceo is with the Department of Medicine, Cooper Medical School of Rowan University, Cooper University Health Care, Camden, NJ. Cordelia Stearns is with High Country Community Health, Boone, NC. Kathleen Shapley-Quinn is with Carolina Advocates for Climate, Health, and Equity, Chapel Hill, NC. Matthew Salzman is with the Department of Emergency and Addiction Medicine, Cooper Medical School of Rowan University, Cooper University Health Care, Camden, NJ.

Hurricane Helene took the mountains of western North Carolina by surprise. As emergency personnel scrambled to mobilize resources, securing medications for patients with opioid use disorder (OUD) was not at the forefront. Yet for "James," who had been stabilized on buprenorphine, the storm's destruction became a life-or-death crisis. Trapped behind a flooded creek with no access to his clinic, he faced a stark choice: withdrawal or use of fentanyl. A community health center in western North Carolina scrambled to open a functional telephone line three days after the storm, anticipating calls from patients looking for water, housing, and oxygen. But overwhelmingly, the calls that poured in were from patients taking buprenorphine, desperate to access their medication as they went into withdrawal.

During Hurricane Helene, several opioid treatment programs (OTPs) in western North Carolina closed for days or weeks as a result of flooding, staff displacement, or power loss. Patients faced road closures, collapsed bridges, and fuel shortages that made travel impossible. Nearly a year later, infrastructure damage continued to impede access to care. Communication failures compounded the crisis: cell towers were down, clinics lost access to health records, and pharmacies often lacked buprenorphine because of disrupted supply chains. Amid competing disaster priorities such as housing, food, and infection control, substance use treatment was deprioritized.[1–3]

Such scenarios are increasingly common as climate-driven disasters expose systemic weaknesses in addiction treatment. Strict regulations, fragile clinical infrastructure, and inadequate emergency planning jeopardize access to methadone and buprenorphine. Even outside of disaster contexts, access to medications for OUD remains far from ideal, with major gaps in availability, affordability, and equity leaving the most vulnerable individuals unreached.

CLIMATE DISASTERS AS A CATALYST FOR OPIOID VULNERABILITY

Public health disasters, including those resulting from climate change, disrupt health services.[4] Opioid misuse often increases after disasters, as heightened stress, loss of community resources, and mental health strain can drive increased drug use.[5,6] Individuals with preexisting mental health conditions are especially vulnerable, turning to substances as coping mechanisms. Disasters also disrupt treatment programs and the medical supply chain, limiting access to opioid therapies and pushing individuals toward illicit substances such as fentanyl.[7,8] These supply shocks amplify overdose risks, particularly when health systems are already strained.

In addition, the economic fallout of natural disasters compounds vulnerability. Economic downturns have been linked to rising drug-related deaths, as weakened labor markets and financial instability exacerbate opioid misuse. Intersecting factors of mental health stressors, treatment disruptions, drug market volatility, and economic decline create conditions where climate-related disasters heighten the risk of opioid use and overdose.

SYSTEMIC GAPS AND INEQUITIES IN DISASTER PREPAREDNESS

The United States health care system is poorly prepared for the rising frequency of climate-related events, with most facilities lacking resilience plans to

AJPH February 2026, Vol. 116, No. 2

ensure continuity of care for chronic conditions such as OUD.[9] Unlike insulin or epinephrine, medications for OUD are controlled substances that cannot easily be stockpiled because of existing regulations, rendering those with OUD reliant on a fragile health care delivery system to avoid withdrawal and relapse.

Climate change also magnifies existing inequalities. Low-income communities, rural residents, and people of color are disproportionately exposed to hazards such as flooding and air pollution while lacking adaptive infrastructure such as reliable housing, transportation, and health care access. For people with OUD, these vulnerabilities are compounded by unstable housing, food insecurity, lack of insurance, and stigma within health care systems. Disasters intensify these barriers. Many cannot evacuate safely, end up in shelters unequipped to manage controlled medications, and experience worsening mental health conditions. Stigma and criminalization further contribute to inequitable responses.

POLICY AND SYSTEMIC GAPS

The current regulatory framework governing OUD treatment in the United States remains rigid and ill suited for the realities of climate-fueled disasters. Federal regulations around methadone, in particular, pose significant challenges. Methadone is available only through federally certified OTPs, which require daily, in-person dosing and impose strict limits on take-home doses. Although federal authorities may issue emergency exceptions during disasters (such as temporary take-home flexibility or relaxed counseling requirements), these measures are inconsistently applied and offer little help if patients cannot reach a facility.

A major barrier is the absence of a standardized interstate system for verifying or transferring treatment records. Pharmacy shortages and prescriber inaccessibility further compound the problem. Preparedness protocols rarely include OUD treatment continuity. Few OTPs maintain disaster-ready infrastructure such as backup power, mobile dosing, or evacuation support, and most public health emergency frameworks omit substance use treatment entirely.

PROMISING PRACTICES AND INNOVATIONS

The COVID-19 pandemic served as an unexpected proving ground for how regulatory flexibility can sustain continuity of care for individuals with OUD during crises.[10] Federal waivers allowing extended take-home methadone doses and buprenorphine initiation via telehealth, including audio-only visits, reduced daily clinic burdens, expanded access in underserved areas, and showed no increase in adverse events, prompting calls for permanent policy adoption (Box 1).[11]

Future preparedness strategies should build on these lessons by improving data sharing and operational flexibility. Expanding prescription drug monitoring programs (PDMPs) to include treatment plans and not just prescriptions could facilitate continuity of care across disrupted systems. In the absence of fully interoperable health records, parallel information-sharing platforms can help clinicians verify treatment history, reduce inequities, and coordinate services more effectively.

Operational innovations also demonstrate promise. Mobile medications for opiate use disorder (MOUD) units deployed after hurricanes and wildfires have provided on-site dosing, reassessments, and harm reduction services such as naloxone and syringe exchange. After Hurricane Helene, such units, paired with peer outreach workers, filled critical gaps when OTPs were inaccessible for weeks. Some health departments now stockpile MOUD alongside traditional emergency supplies, reflecting its essential role (Box 1).

Interdisciplinary collaboration is equally vital.[11] Coordination between emergency medicine teams, addiction specialists, and primary care ensures safe medication transitions, such as transitioning from daily methadone to extended release. Social workers, case managers, and community health workers can help sustain adherence and psychosocial stability, although their own vulnerabilities during disasters highlight the need for supplemental support. To help address this gap, a well-prepared Medical Reserve Corps mobilizing trained volunteers including clinicians, pharmacists, and behavioral health specialists could reinforce continuity of care when local capacity is strained. Interagency communication protocols that enable real-time data sharing and shared care plans are critical for maintaining continuity of care during disasters.

RECOMMENDATIONS

To prevent a "disaster within a disaster," continuity of OUD treatment must be recognized as essential in emergency preparedness. Our recommendations span federal, state, community, health system, and clinical levels. They include codifying emergency flexibilities,

BOX 1— Policy Recommendations to Support Medications for Opiate Use Disorder in Disasters

Level	Domain	Strategy
Federal level	Codify emergency flexibilities	Enable automatic expansion of take-home doses and emergency dosing at alternative sites without requiring federal waivers. Develop preapproved emergency exemptions for disaster-prone states.
	Develop interoperable treatment registries	Establish cross-state systems so that OTPs and providers can verify patient status and transfer care quickly. Link with prescription drug monitoring programs for real-time updates.
	Mandate disaster planning at OTPs	Require federally funded programs to test and maintain emergency continuity protocols, triage protocols (virtually and in-person), and communication drills.
	Integrate MOUD into emergency management systems	Include MOUD logistics and triage alignment within FEMA, DHHS, state, and local emergency operations frameworks.
	Develop MOUD-capable Medical Reserve Corps	Embed MOUD continuity into Medical Reserve Corps preparedness plans, ensuring that trained volunteers can be rapidly deployed to support medication access and patient care when local providers are unable to respond.
	Emergency communications infrastructure	Support OTPs and emergency departments with satellite phones or Starlink connectivity to enable prescribing and record verification when local networks fail.
State level	Centralized MOUD emergency protocols	Create standardized statewide protocols including rapid waiver activation and preapproved take-home dosing.
	Stock disaster kits with MOUD	Just as vaccines and insulin are prioritized, preposition buprenorphine and naloxone in regional emergency stockpiles and make available to shelters, harm reduction teams, and mobile units to serve displaced individuals.
	Create statewide patient registry	Maintain interoperable patient verification databases to allow displaced individuals to access care across counties or states.
	Integrate with emergency operations centers	Embed MOUD continuity into state disaster response plans and coordinate with Medical Reserve Corps, OTPs, hospitals, and harm reduction programs.
Community level	Establish mobile MAT units and pop-up clinics	Deploy mobile MOUD units and medical tents equipped with refrigeration, secure storage, and DEA-compliant protocols.
	Advance planning for helicopter medication drop sites and drone recovery protocols	Identify and preapprove helicopter landing zones for medication dropoffs in rural, mountainous, and flood-prone regions, such as school fields, hospital rooftops, or fire department lots, mapped in coordination with local emergency management agencies and vetted for DEA-compliant storage and handoff procedures. Deployment of drones could support delivering medication to isolated communities but requires advance planning for designated, secure areas where drones can safely land or be retrieved after delivery. Local community health centers or OTP satellites can serve as drone docking stations, equipped with trained staff and secure storage to manage inbound supplies and confirm patient identities.
	Create community outreach network	Train peer navigators, community health workers, and mutual-aid groups to perform patient check-ins and distribute harm reduction supplies during disasters.
	Integrate in shelter protocols	Require shelters to provide secure, private spaces for dosing and storage; coordinate with OTPs for continuity of care.
	Local communication hubs	Equip community health centers with satellite phones or radios to maintain connectivity with OTPs and emergency offices.
Health system level	Emergency communication and data access	Maintain electronic health record connectivity through satellite systems; ensure ability to verify prescriptions and enable telehealth.
	High-risk patient database	Identify patients dependent on time-sensitive treatments (e.g., dialysis, MOUD, ventilators) for proactive outreach.
	Patient communication protocols	Develop automated alerts and scripts to inform patients of weather threats, clinic closures, and alternate dosing sites.
	Occupational and staffing resilience	Stockpile supplies (food, water, fuel) for staff; create flexible staffing models for rapid role reassignment.
Practice level	Provider preparedness and training	Implement training on disaster readiness and MOUD continuity, including telehealth prescribing rules.
	Weather resilience lead	Assign a clinic lead to coordinate emergency planning with local/state agencies and maintain updated staff protocols.
	Continuity drills	Incorporate MOUD continuity into annual emergency drills.
	Patient preparedness education	Counsel patients to maintain naloxone, backup contacts, and awareness of alternate treatment locations.

Note. DEA = Drug Enforcement Administration; DHHS = Department of Health and Human Services; FEMA = Federal Emergency Management Agency; MAT = Medication-Assisted Treatment; MOUD = medications for opiate use disorder; OTP = opioid treatment program.

developing interoperable registries, mandating disaster planning at OTPs, and embedding MOUD into emergency operations. Innovations such as mobile units, harm reduction partnerships, and resilient communication systems further strengthen continuity of care.

If these recommendations are to be operationalized, responsibilities must be defined across all levels of governance and care. Federal agencies including the Substance Abuse and Mental Health Services Administration (SAMHSA), the Drug Enforcement Administration (DEA), and the Department of Health and Human Services (DHHS) should codify emergency flexibilities including preapproved take-home methadone dosing and telehealth buprenorphine initiation, eliminating reliance on ad hoc waivers during disasters. These agencies, which already oversee OTP licensing and security, are well positioned to enforce such standards and allocate funding through mechanisms such as SAMHSA block grants, Federal Emergency Management Agency preparedness funds, and state resilience programs. Medicaid and Medicare could further incentivize compliance by linking reimbursement to verified continuity-of-care plans.

State governments should maintain centralized treatment registries, standardized emergency protocols, and stockpiles of buprenorphine and naloxone alongside other essential medications. Health systems and OTPs must develop, test, and regularly update disaster continuity plans with designated resilience leads. Local agencies, shelters, and community partners should integrate MOUD into shelter operations, ensuring secure storage, dosing, and outreach through peer navigators. Clinicians need training and decision support tools to manage continuity of care in resource-limited settings.

By explicitly delineating these responsibilities from federal policymakers to frontline clinicians, our recommendations outline a coordinated, multilayered approach that could be tailored at the local level. Embedding MOUD into disaster planning requires leadership, accountability, and action across all tiers of the health care and emergency response systems, ensuring that patients with OUD are not left behind during climate-driven crises. AJPH

CORRESPONDENCE

Correspondence should be sent to Elizabeth Cerceo, MD, DCM, Cooper Medical School of Rowan University, 401 Broadway, Camden, NJ 08103 (e-mail: cerceo-elizabeth@cooperhealth.edu). Reprints can be ordered at http://www.ajph.org by clicking the "Reprints" link.

PUBLICATION INFORMATION

Full Citation: Cerceo E, Stearns C, Shapley-Quinn K, Salzman M. Disaster within a disaster: ensuring access to opioid use disorder treatment during natural crises. *Am J Public Health*. 2026;116(2):171–174.

Acceptance Date: November 12, 2025

DOI: https://doi.org/10.2105/AJPH.2025.308354

ORCID iDs:
Elizabeth Cerceo https://orcid.org/0000-0003-3155-2193

Matthew Salzman https://orcid.org/0000-0002-8277-4928

CONTRIBUTORS

E. Cerceo and K. Shapley-Quinn conceived the project. E. Cerceo drafted the initial work and made revisions for important intellectual content. C. Stearns, K. Shapley-Quin, and M. Salzman made substantial contributions to the conception and design of the work.

CONFLICTS OF INTEREST

The authors have no competing interests or disclosures to report.

REFERENCES

1. Lokmic-Tomkins Z, Bhandari D, Bain C, Borda A, Kariotis TC, Reser D. Lessons learned from natural disasters around digital health technologies and delivering quality healthcare. *Int J Environ Res Public Health*. 2023;20(5):4542. https://doi.org/10.3390/ijerph20054542
2. Federal Communications Commission. FCC/FEMA emergency communications tips. Available at: https://www.fcc.gov/emergency. Accessed August 31, 2025.
3. Federal Communications Commission. Communications status report for areas impacted by Hurricane Helene. Available at: https://docs.fcc.gov/public/attachments/DOC-406055A1.pdf. Accessed August 31, 2025.
4. Eisenberg MD, McCourt A, Stuart EA, et al. Studying how state health services delivery policies can mitigate the effects of disasters on drug addiction treatment and overdose: protocol for a mixed-methods study. *PLoS One*. 2021;16(12):e0261115. https://doi.org/10.1371/journal.pone.0261115
5. Charlson F, Ali S, Benmarhnia T, et al. Climate change and mental health: a scoping review. *Int J Environ Res Public Health*. 2021;18(9):4486. https://doi.org/10.3390/ijerph18094486
6. Sharpe I, Davison CM. Climate change, climate-related disasters and mental disorder in low- and middle-income countries: a scoping review. *BMJ Open*. 2021;11(10):e051908. https://doi.org/10.1136/bmjopen-2021-051908
7. Shahzad M, Nogueira LM, Wagner A. Threats of weather disasters for drug manufacturing facilities in the US. *JAMA*. 2025;334(15):1390–1392. https://doi.org/10.1001/jama.2025.13843
8. Woodward CA, Issa FS, Caneva DC, et al. Combating the opioid crisis and its national security threat through CReDO: a multidisciplinary solution with disaster medicine implications. *Disaster Med Public Health Prep*. 2023;17:e509. https://doi.org/10.1017/dmp.2023.173
9. Gkouliaveras V, Kalogiannidis S, Kalfas D, Kontsas S. Effects of climate change on health and health systems: a systematic review of preparedness, resilience, and challenges. *Int J Environ Res Public Health*. 2025;22(2):232. https://doi.org/10.3390/ijerph22020232
10. Russell C, Ali F, Nafeh F, Rehm J, LeBlanc S, Elton-Marshall T. Identifying the impacts of the COVID-19 pandemic on service access for people who use drugs (PWUD): a national qualitative study. *J Subst Abuse Treat*. 2021;129:108374. https://doi.org/10.1016/j.jsat.2021.108374
11. Buchman DZ, Lo S, Ding P, et al. Palliative care for people who use drugs during communicable disease epidemics and pandemics: a scoping review on access, policies, and programs and guidelines. *Palliat Med*. 2023;37(4):426–443. https://doi.org/10.1177/02692163221143153

Roadblocks to Rural Health: State Transportation Policies' Impact on Health Care Access in Virginia's Rural Communities: 2021–2022

Katherine Y. Tossas, PhD, Bianca D. Owens, PhD, Michael O'Grady, MS, Jinlei Zhao, PhD, and Robert A. Winn, MD

Individual and community-level transportation barriers are known drivers of health disparities, especially in rural areas. In a 2021–2022 community-based project to improve cancer screening at federally qualified health centers in Virginia, Department of Transportation policy governing road signage emerged as an unexpected but actionable barrier. Following successful advocacy for road signs directing patients to a rural federally qualified health center, screening rates increased. This highlights the need to recognize unexpected access barriers and engage nontraditional partners, such as transportation agencies, to reduce regulatory-level barriers. (*Am J Public Health*. 2026;116(2):175–179. https://doi.org/10.2105/AJPH.2025.308285)

AJPH February 2026, Vol. 116, No. 2

Individual and community-level transportation barriers impede timely access to health care, particularly among vulnerable and rural populations.[1–4] They contribute to racial and rural cancer disparities,[2,5] affecting stage at detection, access to guideline-concordant care, emergency department visits, survival, and mortality.[2,6,7]

STUDY OBJECTIVE

We present a practice-based observation from a community-based participatory research (CBPR) project involving our academic team, Central Virginia Health Services' Brunswick Health Center (BHC), and a local community organization in Brunswick County, Virginia, to increase colorectal and cervical cancer screening at federally qualified health centers (FQHCs). Although BHC staff knew of long-standing challenges regarding the visibility of its facility, significance as a structural barrier was not apparent to academic partners until they visited. The issue, although familiar to the clinic, was clarified through the CBPR process and collaborative problem solving. The challenge pertained to the Virginia Department of Transportation (VDOT) policy that restricted signage on limited-access highways (i.e., major roads with few intersections, entrances, or exits). BHC sits on an unnamed dirt road branching off a limited-access highway, making it hard to find.

RESEARCH QUESTIONS

We sought to (1) explore the impacts of regulatory transportation barriers on FQHC access locally and statewide, and (2) provide a template for advocacy to potentially increase cancer-screening access via improved visual access to a rural FQHC.

PARTICIPANTS, SAMPLE, GEOGRAPHIC LOCATION, SETTING, AND YEAR OF STUDY

We obtained demographic data from the US Census Bureau and county health rankings, and participating FQHCs reported patient visits and cancer-screening rates using 2019 internal records. BHC is part of a network of 18 clinics that served 45 792 patients in 2019. Of these, 23.5% were uninsured and 28.9% were insured by Medicaid. BHC provides primary care, cancer screening, behavioral health services, and dental services. In 2019, BHC reported that 1568 patients were eligible for colorectal or cervical cancer screening; of these, 25% and 22%, respectively, were screened.

Brunswick County has a high proportion of Black residents (53% vs 20% statewide) as well as twice the state's poverty rate (20.8% vs 10.2%) and an uninsured rate near 10%.[8] BHC was one of five FQHCs participating in Project COALESCE (January 2021–December 2022), a CBPR study pairing FQHCs with local community organizations to identify and address barriers to cancer screening,[9] which is known to be lower among FQHC patients.[10]

Before Project COALESCE, BHC requested—but was denied—an exemption to VDOT policy to install signage directing patients to the clinic. The exemption process itself posed an insurmountable administrative burden: VDOT required a formal petition supported by the town government, an independently commissioned traffic and safety analysis, and legal review to show that boundary changes or exceptions would not conflict with existing statutes. Alternative options included pursuing a statewide regulatory amendment, lobbying for a statutory change through the legislature, and filing litigation—each of which require extensive financial resources, technical expertise, and political capital far beyond the capacity of a small, rural FQHC. Although we conducted Project COALESCE from 2021 to 2022, we used 2019 data as the baseline to reflect typical pre–COVID-19 pandemic screening rates and to avoid 2020 distortions from COVID-19 disruptions.

METHODS

In line with CBPR principles,[11] we collaborated with BHC, community organizations, and other stakeholders to advocate policy change to improve health care and cancer-screening access. We used institutional resources to complete BHC's exemption application and petition to reclassify sections of the nearby highway so that signage could be installed. Goals included catalyzing efforts to create a permanent statutory fix to help other FQHCs avoid the time-consuming exemption request process. This action-oriented approach exemplifies how CBPR can translate community-identified challenges into advocacy efforts. Our advocacy included the following:

- We engaged with a consultant from VDOT to conduct an engineering review and create a report describing BHC, its patient population, and the consequences of diminished facility visibility.
- We approached residents, the town government, and other stakeholders to request letters of support for signage and to describe to them BHC's importance to community health.
- We requested meetings with VDOT and local and state elected officials to explain the issue and garner their support.

Our analytic approach emerged from CBPR discussions in which the issue of directional signage at BHC prompted questions about whether other FQHCs faced similar geospatial barriers. To explore the scope and potential effects of VDOT policy on FQHC access, we obtained address data for all 202 FQHCs and Look-Alikes (i.e., health centers that meet all the requirements to qualify as an FQHC but do not receive the full federal Section 330 grant funding that FQHCs receive) in Virginia from the Health Resources and Services Administration's (HRSA's) 2021 database. This aligned with the project's active period (2021–2022). We geocoded addresses and used ArcGIS (Esri, Redlands, CA) to identify FQHCs located at or within 3200 feet of limited-access highways; this is equivalent to the distance between the index FQHC and the nearest rural highway. This threshold, although not derived from an average or distribution, provided a practical starting point for exploratory spatial comparisons.

Using this criterion, we found that 123 FQHCs (61% of all HRSA-listed centers) were situated at or within 3200 feet of limited-access highways, suggesting that VDOT signage policies may have broad implications beyond BHC. Collectively, these FQHCs serve approximately 239 000 patients. To validate current clinic status, we repeated this analysis using the updated 2023 HRSA database, which identified 56 centers meeting the same proximity threshold. These findings highlight the potential for systemic impact if policy adjustments are pursued.

KEY FINDINGS

We did not observe any statistically significant differences, but affected FQHCs had higher rurality measures (4% vs 1%; $P = .24$) and a slightly lower proportion of Black residents (23% vs 30%; $P = .72$). We observed little variation across other demographic variables. In 2023, approximately 773 365 patients received care at potentially affected FQHCs (Figure 1), demonstrating potential scope of impact.

As a result of advocacy efforts, VDOT agreed to install directional signs reading "Community Health Center" on either side of the highway and issued a permit allowing BHC to place a larger sign in front of the clinic (Figure 2). The small, unnamed road leading from the highway to BHC was given a name to further facilitate access, and VDOT agreed to conduct site surveying. VDOT also screened maps and imagery of

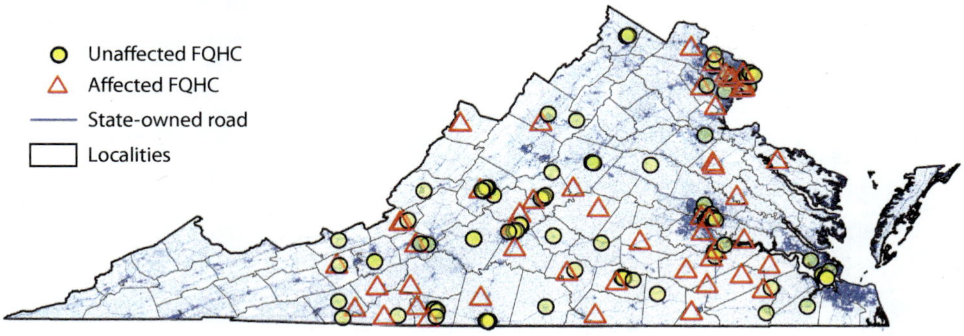

FIGURE 1— Map of State-Owned Roads and FQHCs in Virginia: 2021

Note. FQHC = federally qualified health center. Affected FQHCs (red triangles) are located within 3200 feet of a limited-access highway and potentially affected by Virginia Department of Transportation signage restrictions. Unaffected FQHCs (yellow dots) are located farther than 3200 feet from limited-access highways and are not subject to these restrictions.

other FQHCs statewide to identify similar directional, safety, and visibility challenges (e.g., limited roadway visibility, lack of frontage, complex geometrics, unnamed roads).

EVALUATION, TRANSFERABILITY, AND ADVERSE EFFECTS

At the end of the project (December 2022), after signage installation in January 2022, BHC reported that 1747 patients were eligible for colorectal or cervical cancer screening, up from 1568 in 2019. Of these, 1228 were screened, representing postintervention screening rates of 69% for colorectal cancer and 71% for cervical cancer. This reflects 44- and 49-percentage point increases over the 2019 baseline rates of 25% and 22%. Although we cannot establish causality, clinic staff attributed this improvement partly to improved visibility and strengthened partnerships with community organizations developed through the project.

BHC's permit to install directional signage is a notable victory, with VDOT's commitment to investigate other health care facilities that may benefit from exemptions or zoning changes. Although cancer screening increased after signage installation, we cannot establish causality or rule out other factors—such as community outreach, staff changes, or unrelated health policy shifts—that may explain these changes. Although further research is needed, state-level solutions could include modifying VDOT policy to

a b

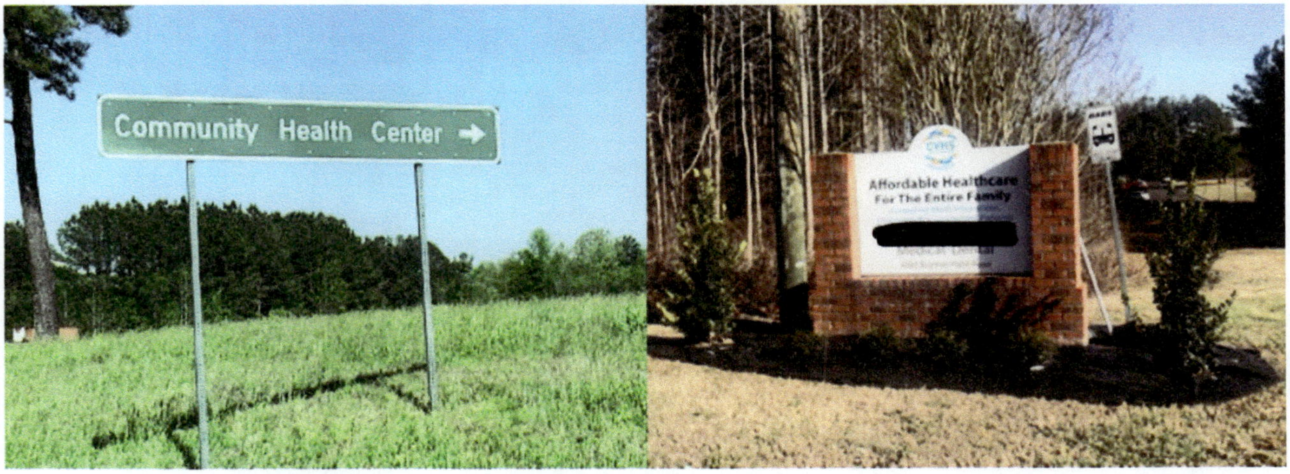

FIGURE 2— Directional Signage Installed by the Virginia Department of Transportation on a Limited-Access Highway Near Federally Qualified Health Centers: Brunswick County, VA, January 2022

Source. Photos courtesy of a community member.

AJPH February 2026, Vol. 116, No. 2

exempt health care facilities from signage restrictions and simplifying exception processes. The most sustainable approaches involve cross-sector collaborations[12] to align transportation and health policy, such as joint task forces consisting of VDOT, health and local government officials, FQHCs, clinicians, patients, public health professionals, and other stakeholders. Community-engaged research partnerships could provide data-driven insights into transportation design that support local health and cancer care needs.

When unexpected barriers arise, CBPR researchers should remain flexible and curious, and they should collaborate with communities to address them.[11] Policymakers should consider similar barriers in their communities and identify opportunities for cross-sector change.[13] Health care facilities should consider potential navigational or facility visibility issues and how they might be remedied. Advocates can bolster signage petitions with letters of endorsements from local governments, FQHC staff and patients, and engineering safety data.

SCALABILITY

Transportation barriers often vary by community context.[14] This case, however, highlights an overlooked barrier that disproportionately affects rural FQHC patients. The partnership successfully removed a significant obstacle through multisectoral collaboration. This approach is key to reducing structural health care access barriers and improving public health. The advocacy and partnership model offers a replicable framework. Future qualitative research could explore traditional and nontraditional transportation barriers—such as signage policies and wayfinding challenges—and inform collaborative disparity reduction. Quantitative work with affected FQHCs is needed to assess signage effects. Research and interventions that identify nontraditional transportation and other barriers and develop tailored solutions with local and state agencies (e.g., transportation agencies) may help reduce cancer disparities in other communities.

PUBLIC HEALTH SIGNIFICANCE

FQHCs play a critical role in reducing cancer disparities[15]; however, their impact depends on resolving access barriers, including findability, transportation, appointment availability, affordability, and care coordination. This case shows how transportation agencies influence health care access. Cross-sector collaboration can mitigate policy barriers and improve outcomes. Transportation policy—including that on signage and public transit—is a public health issue.[13,14] Achieving healthy communities requires aligning infrastructure with health care access goals. AJPH

ABOUT THE AUTHORS

Katherine Y. Tossas is an assistant professor in the School of Public Health, Department of Social and Behavioral Sciences, and the director of the Office of Catchment Area Data Analytics, Massey Comprehensive Cancer Center, Virginia Commonwealth University, Richmond, VA. Bianca D. Owens is a postdoctoral research fellow at Massey Comprehensive Cancer Center. Michael O'Grady is a doctoral candidate with the L. Douglas Wilder School of Government and Public Affairs, Virginia Commonwealth University. Jinlei Zhao is a research specialist in the Office of Catchment Area Data Analytics. Robert A. Winn is the director of Massey Comprehensive Cancer Center.

CORRESPONDENCE

Correspondence should be sent to Katherine Y. Tossas, 401 College St, Richmond, VA 23298 (e-mail: tossask@vcu.edu). Reprints can be ordered at https://www.ajph.org by clicking the "Reprints" link.

PUBLICATION INFORMATION

Full Citation: Tossas KY, Owens BD, O'Grady M, Zhao J, Winn RA. Roadblocks to rural health: state transportation policies' impact on health care access in Virginia's rural communities: 2021–2022. *Am J Public Health*. 2026;116(2):175–179.

Acceptance Date: August 26, 2025.

DOI: https://doi.org/10.2105/AJPH.2025.308285

ORCID iDs:

Katherine Y. Tossas https://orcid.org/0000-0001-6872-2294

Bianca D. Owens https://orcid.org/0000-0002-7983-0298

Jinlei Zhao https://orcid.org/0000-0003-0866-5026

Robert A. Winn https://orcid.org/0000-0001-5948-9291

CONTRIBUTORS

K. Y. Tossas conceptualized and prepared the first draft of the article, acquired funding, and administered the project. K. Y. Tossas, B. D. Owens, and J. Zhao reviewed and edited the article and developed the methodology. K. Y. Tossas, M. O'Grady, and J. Zhao formally analyzed the data. M. O'Grady and J. Zhao curated the data. R. A. Winn provided supervision and senior support. All authors read and agreed to the published version of the article.

ACKNOWLEDGMENTS

This project is funded by Pfizer (global medical grant 63713541) and overseen by the American Cancer Society.

The authors would like to acknowledge the contributions of Teya Whitehead, Vanessa B. Sheppard, and the participating federally qualified health centers, community organizations, and community members.

Note. The funders had no role in the design of the study; the collection, analyses, or interpretation of data; the writing of the article, or the decision to publish the results.

CONFLICTS OF INTEREST

The authors have no conflicts of interest to declare.

HUMAN PARTICIPANT PROTECTION

Ethical review and approval were waived for this study because as a quality improvement initiative, it is not considered research or intended to produce generalizable outcomes beyond those applicable to participating entities. The intent is to suggest potentially effective models, strategies, and assessment tools or provide benchmarks rather than to develop or contribute to generalizable knowledge.

REFERENCES

1. Syed ST, Gerber BS, Sharp LK. Traveling towards disease: transportation barriers to health care access. *J Community Health*. 2013;38(5):976–993. https://doi.org/10.1007/s10900-013-9681-1
2. Zahnd WE, Murphy C, Knoll M, et al. The intersection of rural residence and minority race/ethnicity in cancer disparities in the United States. *Int J Environ Res Public Health*. 2021;18(4):1384. https://doi.org/10.3390/ijerph18041384
3. Peipins LA, Graham S, Young R, Lewis B, Flanagan B. Racial disparities in travel time to radiotherapy facilities in the Atlanta metropolitan area. *Soc Sci Med*. 2013;89:32–38. https://doi.org/10.1016/j.socscimed.2013.04.018
4. Wercholuk AN, Parikh AA, Snyder RA. The road less traveled: transportation barriers to cancer care delivery in the rural patient population. *JCO Oncol Pract*. 2022;18(9):652–662. https://doi.org/10.1200/op.22.00122
5. Singh GK, Williams SD, Siahpush M, Mulhollen A. Socioeconomic, rural–urban, and racial inequalities in US cancer mortality: part I—all cancers and lung cancer and part II—colorectal, prostate, breast, and cervical cancers. *J Cancer Epidemiol*. 2011;2011(1):107497. https://doi.org/10.1155/2011/107497
6. Jiang C, Yabroff KR, Deng L, et al. Transportation barriers, emergency room use, and mortality risk among US adults by cancer history. *J Natl Cancer Inst*. 2023;115(7):815–821. https://doi.org/10.1093/jnci/djad050
7. Ambroggi M, Biasini C, Del Giovane C, Fornari F, Cavanna L. Distance as a barrier to cancer diagnosis and treatment: review of the literature. *Oncologist*. 2015;20(12):1378–1385. https://doi.org/10.1634/theoncologist.2015-0110
8. US Census Bureau. Brunswick County, VA: profile data. Available at: https://censusreporter.org/profiles/05000US51025-brunswick-county-va. Accessed September 13, 2023.
9. Tossas KY, Reitzel S, Schifano K, et al. Project COALESCE—an example of academic institutions as conveners of community–clinic partnerships to improve cancer screening access. *Int J Environ Res Public Health*. 2022;19(2):957. https://doi.org/10.3390/ijerph19020957
10. Amboree TL, Montealegre JR, Parker SL, et al. National breast, cervical, and colorectal cancer screening use in federally qualified health centers. *JAMA Intern Med*. 2024;184(6):671–679. https://doi.org/10.1001/jamainternmed.2024.0693
11. Minkler M. Community-based research partnerships: challenges and opportunities. *J Urban Health*. 2005;82(suppl 2):ii3–ii12. https://doi.org/10.1093/jurban/jti034
12. Cantilina K, Daly SR, Reed MP, Hampshire RC. Approaches and barriers to addressing equity in transportation: experiences of transportation practitioners. *Transp Res Rec*. 2021;2675(10):972–985. https://doi.org/10.1177/03611981211014533
13. Ingram M, Leih R, Adkins A, Sonmez E, Yetman E. Health disparities, transportation equity and complete streets: a case study of a policy development process through the lens of critical race theory. *J Urban Health*. 2020;97(6):876–886. https://doi.org/10.1007/s11524-020-00460-8
14. Combs TS, Shay E, Salvesen D, Kolosna C, Madeley M. Understanding the multiple dimensions of transportation disadvantage: the case of rural North Carolina. *Case Stud Transp Policy*. 2016;4(2):68–77. https://doi.org/10.1016/j.cstp.2016.02.004
15. Adams SA, Choi SK, Khang L, et al. Decreased cancer mortality-to-incidence ratios with increased accessibility of federally qualified health centers. *J Community Health*. 2015;40(4):633–641. https://doi.org/10.1007/s10900-014-9978-8

Reassessing Medicaid's Protective Effect During Continuous-Coverage Unwinding: A Focused Reanalysis and Practice Note

Shiya Zeng, PhD, Shi Huang, PhD, Wenjing Chen, PhD, and Ruixiang Li, PhD

ABOUT THE AUTHORS

Shiya Zeng, Shi Huang, Wenjing Chen, and Ruixiang Li are with the Clinical Medical College, Southwest Medical University, Luzhou, Sichuan, China.

Han et al. report slower mortality growth in Medicaid expansion than nonexpansion states during 2018 to 2022, reinforcing a population-level protective effect of coverage expansion.[1,2] We propose a focused extension: after the COVID-19 public health emergency, states began "unwinding"—resuming routine eligibility renewals and terminations for millions who remained continuously enrolled.[3] We hypothesize that unwinding may erode this protection through coverage churn among patients needing uninterrupted medications and outpatient care. We define it as the state-led return to regular redeterminations and associated disenrollments after continuous coverage ended.[3]

Early data from community networks and multistate reports show measurable coverage loss during unwinding—especially among children—with disparities by age, sex, race/ethnicity, and medical complexity.[4,5] These patterns align with pathways by which churn interrupts prescriptions (e.g., insulin, asthma controller inhalers) and triggers avoidable acute events; other high-need domains include mental health, substance use disorders, and HIV care.[4–6] To test whether this protective effect is being offset, we suggest re-estimating the Han et al. models with 2023 through 2025 data and an explicit unwinding period.[1]

Analytically, we recommend three additions to the difference-in-differences framework: (1) county-level vulnerability stratification (rurality, social vulnerability indices, Tribal lands, racial/ethnic composition) to capture geographic heterogeneity in mortality[6]; (2) near-real-time proxy outcomes—monthly pharmacy refill gaps, emergency department visits, and 30-day readmissions for asthma or diabetes complications; and (3) policy-timed breakpoints aligned with state calendars and Centers for Medicare and Medicaid Services (CMS) waiver flexibilities to separate clinical effects from procedural disenrollments.[3] These refinements are feasible and consistent with previous evidence published in *AJPH* on structural vulnerability and pandemic-era mortality gradients.[6]

For policy and practice, much activity has occurred since 2023. Managed care organizations and community health centers expanded renewal outreach, portal and text message refill reminders, and bridge refills; CMS disseminated unwinding toolkits; advocacy groups (e.g., Health Care for All) provided renewal assistance and coverage retention; and independent state dashboards (e.g., KFF) document renewal outcomes and procedural terminations.[5] States should publish monthly county-level churn dashboards—including disenrollment, successful redetermination, and reinstatement rates—to guide outreach and minimize treatment interruptions.[5]

Finally, threats to Medicaid coverage extend beyond unwinding. The 2025 federal budget reconciliation law contains large health-spending reductions; the Congressional Budget Office estimates more than $900 billion in Medicaid cuts (more than $1 trillion in total health cuts) over 10 years and increases in the uninsured, which could compound postunwinding disruptions in coverage and access.[7] These headwinds underscore the urgency of stabilizing eligibility and reducing churn, particularly for children and other high-need populations. AJPH

CORRESPONDENCE

Correspondence should be sent to Ruixiang Li, 319 Zhongshan Rd, Luzhou, Sichuan 646000, China (e-mail: liruixiang2025@163.com). Reprints can be ordered at https://www.ajph.org by clicking the "Reprints" link.

PUBLICATION INFORMATION

Full Citation: Zeng S, Huang S, Chen W, Li R. Reassessing Medicaid's protective effect during continuous-coverage unwinding: a focused reanalysis and practice note. *Am J Public Health*. 2026;116(2):180–181.

Acceptance Date: October 22, 2025.

DOI: https://doi.org/10.2105/AJPH.2025.308346

ORCID iDs:
Shi Huang https://orcid.org/0009-0005-4796-0660

Wenjing Chen https://orcid.org/0009-0007-6500-1943

Ruixiang Li https://orcid.org/0009-0008-3553-2951

CONTRIBUTORS

S. Zeng, S. Huang, and W. Chen contributed equally to data collection, analysis, and article drafting. R. Li originated the study, supervised the research process, and critically revised the article.

CONFLICTS OF INTEREST

The authors report no conflicts of interest.

REFERENCES

1. Han X, Shi KS, Fan Q, Choudhury PP, Hu X, Yabroff KR. Medicaid expansion and US mortality rates during the COVID-19 pandemic, 2018–2022. *Am J Public Health.* 2025;115(6):890–899. https://doi.org/10.2105/AJPH.2025.308045
2. Allen H. Does Medicaid improve health? *Am J Public Health.* 2025;115(6):833–834. https://doi.org/10.2105/AJPH.2025.308124
3. Centers for Medicare & Medicaid Services. Unwinding and returning to regular operations after COVID-19. Available at: https://www.medicaid.gov/resources-for-states/coronavirus-disease-2019-covid-19/unwinding-and-returning-regular-operations-after-covid-19. Accessed September 22, 2025.
4. Bensken WP, Dankovchik J, Fein HL, Duhon G, Sills MR. Unwinding of continuous Medicaid coverage among pediatric community health center patients. *JAMA Netw Open.* 2025;8(2):e2458155. https://doi.org/10.1001/jamanetworkopen.2024.58155
5. KFF. Medicaid enrollment and unwinding tracker. 2025. Available at: https://www.kff.org/medicaid/medicaid-enrollment-and-unwinding-tracker. Accessed September 22, 2025.
6. Riley AR, Kim YJ, Flores Morales J, Charpignon ML, DeVost MA, Chen YH. Inequities in excess pandemic mortality among documented and undocumented immigrants in California, 2020–2023. *Am J Public Health.* 2025;115(10):1681–1690. https://doi.org/10.2105/AJPH.2025.308150
7. Congressional Budget Office. Estimated budgetary effects of Public Law 119–21, to provide for reconciliation pursuant to Title II of H. Con. Res. 14, relative to the budget enforcement baseline for consideration in the Senate. Congressional Budget Office report. July 21, 2025. Available at: https://www.cbo.gov/publication/61569. Accessed September 22, 2025.

Use of an Inappropriate Control Period When Exploring the Impacts of Cannabis Legalization

Bobby P. Smyth, MRCPsych, PhD, and Peter McCarron, MRCPsych, PhD

ABOUT THE AUTHORS

Bobby P. Smyth is with the Institute of Population Health, Trinity College Dublin, Dublin, Ireland, and HSE Addiction Services, Cherry Orchard Hospital, Dublin. Peter McCarron is with HSE Addiction Services, Cherry Orchard Hospital, Dublin, Ireland.

See also Myran et al., p. 183.

In their article on cannabis-related hospitalizations across 2015 to 2022, Myran et al. make the strong conclusion that "legalization in Canada was associated with reductions in cannabis-related hospitalizations for youths below the [minimum legal age]."[1(p1166)] This conclusion seems excessive. It could cause policymakers globally to think that a move from prohibition to legalization may yield health benefits for children and adolescents.

It is not appropriate to use the years 2015 to 2018 as the control "preintervention" period. This was a legalization preparation phase, a part of the legalization process.[2] Arguably, there was de facto legalization in place during this time. There was a tolerated and steadily expanding network of cannabis dispensaries operating in an unregulated gray market. In May 2016, the mayor of Toronto described the issue as "verging on being out of control."[3] These dispensaries served as a major source of cannabis for youths before legalization.[4] This important context is omitted by the authors.

The societal approach to cannabis shifted in Canada about a decade before legalization. The cannabis arrest rate declined incrementally from 2011 despite increases in the prevalence of heavy cannabis use.[5] The authors neglect to mention the fact that laws regarding "medical" cannabis were greatly relaxed in 2014 and the government declared its intention to fully legalize adult use in late 2015.[2,6]

In one of their other recent articles, the authors appropriately described 2015 to September 2018 as the period of "cannabis liberalization," and they demonstrated increasing emergency department attendance relative to a 2010 to 2014 control period.[6] This policy liberalization likely contributed to the rapidly escalating health harms reported in this study and artificially inflated the counterfactual estimates used by the authors in their comparisons.

Readers should also note that Canadian adolescents were global outliers in terms of cannabis use and related health harm well before formal legalization, so the findings from Canada may translate poorly to other settings.[7]

A final key omission by the authors relates to the impact of legalization on children younger than 15 years. Their own past research and that of others indicates significant increases in cannabis-related hospitalizations in that demographic.[5] In an article addressing legalization and youths, that certainly deserved mention. AJPH

CORRESPONDENCE

Correspondence should be sent to Bobby P. Smyth, MRCPsych, PhD, Department of Public Health & Primary Care, Institute of Population Health, Trinity College Dublin, Russell Building, Tallaght Cross West, Dublin 24, Ireland (e-mail: smythbo@tcd.ie). Reprints can be ordered at https://www.ajph.org by clicking the "Reprints" link.

PUBLICATION INFORMATION

Full Citation: Smyth BP, McCarron P. Use of an inappropriate control period when exploring the impacts of cannabis legalization. *Am J Public Health*. 2026;116(2):182–183.

Acceptance Date: October 2, 2025.

DOI: https://doi.org/10.2105/AJPH.2025.308307

ORCID iDs:
Bobby P. Smyth https://orcid.org/0000-0003-3797-5541

Peter McCarron https://orcid.org/0000-0002-4367-035X

CONTRIBUTORS

B. P. Smyth led on the conception of the work. The authors contributed equally to the analysis and the drafting of the work.

ACKNOWLEDGMENTS

The views expressed do not necessarily reflect those of the authors' employers.

CONFLICTS OF INTEREST

The authors have no conflicts of interest to declare.

REFERENCES

1. Myran DT, Talarico R, Pacula RL, et al. Minimum legal age of nonmedical cannabis purchase laws and cannabis-related hospitalizations in Canada, 2015 to 2022. *Am J Public Health*. 2025;115(7): 1166–1174. https://doi.org/10.2105/AJPH.2025.308090
2. Smyth BP, McCarron P. Increase in cannabis-related emergency department presentations in the period immediately before legalization requires explanation. *Addiction*. 2023;118(5): 979–980. https://doi.org/10.1111/add.16128
3. CBC News. Medical marijuana dispensaries "verging on being out of control," Mayor John Tory says. May 6, 2016. Available at: https://www.cbc.ca/news/canada/toronto/tory-medical-marijuana-1.3570263. Accessed September 6, 2025.

4. Hawke LD, Henderson J. Legalization of cannabis use in Canada: impacts on the cannabis use profiles of youth seeking services for substance use. J Subst Abuse Treat. 2021;126:108340. https://doi.org/10.1016/j.jsat.2021.108340
5. Hall W, Stjepanović D, Dawson D, Leung J. The implementation and public health impacts of cannabis legalization in Canada: a systematic review. *Addiction.* 2023;118(11):2062–2072. https://doi.org/10.1111/add.16274
6. Myran DT, Gaudreault A, Pugliese M, Tanuseputro P, Saunders N. Cannabis-involvement in emergency department visits for self-harm following medical and non-medical cannabis legalization. *J Affect Disord.* 2024;351:853–862. https://doi.org/10.1016/j.jad.2024.01.264
7. Smyth BP, Cannon M. Cannabis legalization and adolescent cannabis use: explanation of paradoxical findings. *J Adolesc Health.* 2021;69(1):14–15. https://doi.org/10.1016/j.jadohealth.2021.02.025

Myran et al. Respond

Daniel T. Myran, MD, MPH, Rosalie Pacula, PhD, and Monica Taljaard, PhD

ABOUT THE AUTHORS

Daniel T. Myran is with the Department of Family Medicine, Faculty of Medicine, University of Ottawa, Ottawa, Ontario, Canada. Rosalie Pacula is with the Sol Price School of Public Policy and Schaeffer Center for Health Policy and Economics, University of Southern California, Los Angeles. Monica Taljaard is with the Clinical Epidemiology Program, Ottawa Hospital Research Institute, Ottawa, Ontario, Canada.

See also Smyth and McCarron, p. 182.

We thank Smyth and McCarron for their comments on our recent article, which provide us the opportunity to clarify possible misinterpretations of our results.

First, they suggest that the conclusion of our article is that legalization reduces cannabis harms among young people. This is not what we examined in our study or the conclusion that we intended. Our purpose was to examine whether restrictions on the minimum legal age (MLA) of cannabis purchase are effective in protecting youths below the MLA from cannabis-related hospitalizations. As we indicated, hospitalizations related to cannabis were increasing before legalization among both individuals above and below the MLA. The empirical question we addressed was whether legalization differentially affected the preperiod trend for those below versus above the MLA restrictions, and we observed protective effects for those below the MLA. The appropriate interpretation of our results is that in regions that pursue legalization, MLA restrictions appear to function as intended, preventing legal access and offering some protections to those below the age threshold versus those who can access the legal market. Our study does not suggest, nor do we propose, that jurisdictions should legalize cannabis to reduce youth cannabis use or harms.

Second, they suggest that not examining hospitalizations among very young children, which are primarily accidental child poisonings, is a critical omission of our study. Although we have published separately on large increases in unintentional cannabis poisonings among children,[1,2] these outcomes are not relevant to an analysis of the effectiveness of MLA restrictions for cannabis purchase, as the purpose of our study was not to assess the overall effects of legalization but instead to examine a specific policy element. An appropriate comparison of MLA restrictions is people who are just above or below the MLA, not toddlers and young children who do not intend to consume cannabis or do not have the ability or desire to purchase it.

Third, they argue that 2015 to 2018 was an inappropriate preintervention period because hospitalizations were increasing rapidly in the lead up to legalization, likely as a result of increasing access and changing social norms. We have previously addressed a very similar comment from Smyth and McCarron in further detail, which readers may find helpful.[3] Although we began our study in 2015 because that is when pan-Canadian data on hospitalizations became available, we and others have shown that cannabis-related harms in Canada were increasing before 2015, and the increases observed between 2015 and 2018 were not an anomaly.[4] Our analytical design explicitly accounted for preintervention trends in both the exposed and control groups with respect to evaluating the effectiveness of MLA restrictions. We also disagree that the presence of medical cannabis, a gray cannabis market, and changing social norms in Canada means that our findings will not generalize to other countries as these features are present in many other regions of the world.[5]

Cannabis legalization can encompass a wide spectrum of policy models, and the impacts of legalization will vary across jurisdictions on several factors such as baseline rates of cannabis use and harms and how legalization is implemented (e.g., commercialization or strict public health–oriented regulations). Variations in both implementation and changes in use and health effects have been well documented in Canada.[1,2,6] The main contribution of our study is providing evidence on the effectiveness of MLA restrictions. We conclude that MLAs can be an important public health safeguard in jurisdictions that proceed with legalization; we do not say that they eliminate risks to youths entirely. However, our study suggests that setting a higher MLA (e.g., 21 years instead of 19 years) may offer further benefits by covering a greater number of young people. AJPH

CORRESPONDENCE

Correspondence should be sent to Daniel T. Myran, MD, MPH, Ottawa Hospital Research Institute, 1053 Carling Ave, Box 693, Ottawa, Ontario, K1Y 4E9 Canada (e-mail: dmyran@ohri.ca). Reprints can be ordered at https://www.ajph.org by clicking the "Reprints" link.

PUBLICATION INFORMATION

Full Citation: Myran DT, Pacula R, Taljaard M. Myran et al. respond. *Am J Public Health*. 2026;116(2):183–184.

Acceptance Date: November 4, 2025.

DOI: https://doi.org/10.2105/AJPH.2025.308345

ORCID iDs:
Daniel T. Myran https://orcid.org/0000-0002-8038-300X

Rosalie Pacula https://orcid.org/0000-0002-6145-9865

CONTRIBUTORS

All of the authors made substantial contributions to the concept, design, drafting, and critical revision of the work.

CONFLICTS OF INTEREST

The authors have no conflicts of interest to disclose.

REFERENCES

1. Myran DT, Tanuseputro P, Auger N, Konikoff L, Talarico R, Finkelstein Y. Pediatric hospitalizations for unintentional cannabis poisonings and all-cause poisonings associated with edible cannabis product legalization and sales in Canada. *JAMA Health Forum*. 2023;4(1):e225041. https://doi.org/10.1001/JAMAHEALTHFORUM.2022.5041
2. Myran DT, Tanuseputro P, Auger N, Konikoff L, Talarico R, Finkelstein Y. Edible cannabis legalization and unintentional poisonings in children. *N Engl J Med*. 2022;387(8):757–759. https://doi.org/10.1056/NEJMC2207661
3. Myran DT, Pugliese M, Tanuseputro P, Taljaard M. Response to Smyth & McCarron: Increases in cannabis-attributable emergency department visits during different phases of the pre- and post-legalization period are multi-factorial. *Addiction*. 2023;118(5):980–982. https://doi.org/10.1111/add.16152
4. Zygmunt A, Tanuseputro P, Brown C, Lima I, Rhodes E, Myran D. Changes in rates of hospitalizations due to cannabis harms in Ontario, Canada before the legalization of nonmedical cannabis: retrospective population-level study between 2003 and 2017. *J Addict Med*. 2022;16(3):E177–E184. https://doi.org/10.1097/ADM.0000000000000906
5. United Nations Office of Drugs and Crime. Drug market trends of cannabis and opioids. Available at: https://www.unodc.org/unodc/en/data-and-analysis/wdr-2022_booklet-3.html. Accessed October 2, 2025.
6. Myran DT, Imtiaz S, Konikoff L, Douglas L, Elton-Marshall T. Changes in health harms due to cannabis following legalisation of non-medical cannabis in Canada in context of cannabis commercialisation: a scoping review. *Drug Alcohol Rev*. 2023;42(2):277–298. https://doi.org/10.1111/dar.13546

Reconsidering Conservative Exclusion Criteria in Claims-Based Research on Gender-Affirming Surgery

Rebecca Sanaeikia, MA

ABOUT THE AUTHOR

Rebecca Sanaeikia is a PhD student in the Department of Philosophy, University of Rochester, Rochester, NY.

See also Babbs et al., p. 186.

Babbs et al.[1] provide valuable methodological guidance for claims-based research on gender-affirming surgery among transgender and gender-diverse (TGD) populations. However, I identify a concerning contradiction between their inclusive definition of gender-affirming care and their recommended conservative exclusion criteria that warrants further discussion. The authors define gender-affirming care as "procedures or medications that align physical gender expression with a person's intrinsic gender identity" and acknowledge that cisgender individuals also utilize such care. Yet their methodology systematically excludes cases with concurrent non–gender-specific diagnoses, such as cancer, potentially removing both cisgender individuals and TGD people who receive procedures for mixed clinical reasons.

This exclusion becomes particularly concerning in light of the current hostile political climate.[2] With ongoing legal threats targeting TGD youths[3] and adults accessing gender-affirming care, patients may choose not to disclose their TGD identity or prefer not to be identified as such in a data set labeled as TGD data to protect their privacy and safety. The conservative approach, although well-intentioned, excludes these vulnerable individuals, perpetuating what philosophers term "testimonial silencing," which is the epistemic harm occurring when marginalized individuals cannot disclose their identity because they anticipate negative consequences.[4,5]

Instead, I propose a methodological shift from identifying TGD patients to identifying procedures useful for TGD populations. This approach would include cases in which gender-affirming motivations might exist alongside other clinical justifications, ensuring that research remains relevant to TGD communities without requiring explicit TGD identification. Such an inclusive methodology also enhances data safety by redirecting algorithmic focus from patient identification to procedure classification, reducing potential surveillance risks for vulnerable populations. This reframing acknowledges the complex realities of health care navigation in politically hostile environments while avoiding epistemic harms. By studying data useful for understanding gender-affirming care access patterns rather than definitively categorizing patient identities, researchers can produce knowledge that serves TGD communities without inadvertently contributing to their surveillance or exclusion.

The authors' framework represents important progress in TGD health research methodology. However, given the current political context and safety concerns facing TGD individuals, I encourage researchers to consider more inclusive approaches that capture the full spectrum of gender-affirming care utilization while protecting vulnerable populations from potential harm through research participation. AJPH

CORRESPONDENCE

Correspondence should be sent to Rebecca Sanaeikia, Department of Philosophy, University of Rochester—River Campus, 136 East Squire Dr, Rochester, NY 14623 (e-mail: becca.sanaeikia@rochester.edu). Reprints can be ordered at https://www.ajph.org by clicking the "Reprints" link.

PUBLICATION INFORMATION

Full Citation: Sanaeikia R. Reconsidering conservative exclusion criteria in claims-based research on gender-affirming surgery. *Am J Public Health.* 2026;116(2):185–186.

Acceptance Date: October 10, 2025.

DOI: https://doi.org/10.2105/AJPH.2025.308321

ORCID iD:
Rebecca Sanaeikia https://orcid.org/0009-0006-2158-2654

ACKNOWLEDGMENTS

I want to thank the authors of the original article for their careful contribution to a timely topic.

CONFLICTS OF INTEREST

The author has no conflicts of interest to disclose.

REFERENCES

1. Babbs G, Dai D, Boskey ER, Balkan E, Hughto JMW. Challenges and best practices using claims data to study gender-affirming surgery in transgender and gender-diverse populations. *Am J Public Health.* 2025;115(10):1605–1610. https://doi.org/10.2105/AJPH.2025.308187
2. Trans Legislation Tracker. 2025 anti-trans bills tracker. Available at: https://translegislation.com. Accessed September 27, 2025.
3. Cameron C. Trump officials demanded confidential data about transgender children seeking care. *New York Times.* August 21, 2025. Available at: https://www.nytimes.com/2025/08/20/us/politics/trump-transgender-children-care-subpoena.html. Accessed September 27, 2025.
4. Alpert AB, Babbs G, Sanaeikia R, et al. Doing justice: ethical considerations identifying and researching transgender and gender diverse people in insurance claims data. *J Med Syst.* 2024;48(1):96. https://doi.org/10.1007/s10916-024-02111-w
5. Dotson K. Tracking epistemic violence, tracking practices of silencing. *Hypatia.* 2011;26(2):236–257. https://doi.org/10.1111/j.1527-2001.2011.01177.x

Babbs et al. Respond

Gray Babbs, MPH, Dannie Dai, BA, Elizabeth R. Boskey, PhD, MPH, MSW, Em Balkan, MSW, and Jaclyn M. W. Hughto, PhD, MPH

ABOUT THE AUTHORS

Gray Babbs, Em Balkan, and Jaclyn M. W. Hughto are with the Brown University School of Public Health, Providence, RI. Dannie Dai is with the Boston Health Care for the Homeless Program, Boston, MA. Elizabeth R. Boskey is with Boston Children's Hospital, Boston, MA.

See also Sanaeikia, p. 185.

We thank the author(s) for their thoughtful response and critique (p. 185). We agree that minimizing harm to transgender and gender-diverse (TGD) populations must be a central priority in research. However, it is important to recognize that harm can be conceptualized in multiple, sometimes competing, ways. While the letter noted the risk of testimonial silencing,[1] our approach prioritizes minimizing harm from potential overestimation of TGD medical utilization and centers the importance of analyzing health outcomes of TGD populations as their own, rather than extrapolating from primarily cisgender population data.

To accomplish our goals, we focus on procedures generally recognized by patients, health care professionals, and payers as gender-affirming and performed specifically for gender affirmation. This approach is intentionally conservative. While it inevitably excludes some gender-affirming procedures, it also has several advantages:

1. Respecting intent and avoiding assumptions: If a procedure was not billed as gender-affirming, we are mindful that the patient or provider may not want it to be interpreted that way. For instance, someone undergoing a mastectomy because of cancer may or may not experience it as gender-affirming regardless of their gender identity.
2. Prioritizing TGD population data: Coding for gender-affirming procedures is not particularly specific.[2] Some of the most widely used gender-affirmation procedures and procedure codes are also used for cisgender populations—and the data from cisgender patients would render TGD populations[3] a minority in the data, with outcomes extrapolated from primarily cisgender patients.
3. Focusing on core care areas: Classifying all instances of the more than 700 procedure codes[4] we have identified as *potentially* gender-affirming risks obscuring actual trends in care and can lead to inaccurate conclusions, including, but not limited to, contributing to oversimplified narratives about the rate of gender-affirming procedures.[5,6]

Our research methods are designed to address questions about access to care within a health care system where access is structured around insurance coverage availability. Our methods also reflect our ethical commitment to minimizing harm that could result from a substantial overestimation of the amount—and therefore cost—of gender-affirming care.[7]

More qualitative work is urgently needed to develop a greater understanding of how TGD people conceptualize gender-affirming care, weigh different forms of harm, and want their experiences represented in research. Additional perspectives are essential to improving our understanding of gender-affirming care within an ethical framework that prioritizes the needs and rights of TGD populations. AJPH

CORRESPONDENCE

Correspondence should be sent to Gray Babbs, 121 S Main St, Providence, RI 02906 (e-mail: gray_babbs@brown.edu). Reprints can be ordered at https://www.ajph.org by clicking the "Reprints" link.

PUBLICATION INFORMATION

Full Citation: Babbs G, Dai D, Boskey ER, Balkan E, Hughto JMW. Babbs et al. respond. *Am J Public Health.* 2026;116(2):186–187.

Acceptance Date: November 15, 2025.

DOI: https://doi.org/10.2105/AJPH.2025.308363

ORCID iDs:

Gray Babbs https://orcid.org/0000-0003-4060-571X

Elizabeth R. Boskey https://orcid.org/0000-0002-4982-1323

Em Balkan https://orcid.org/0009-0001-0333-9312

Jaclyn M. W. Hughto https://orcid.org/0000-0003-4722-8179

CONTRIBUTORS

All authors contributed to the conceptualization, drafting, and revising of the work and provided final approval for publication.

CONFLICTS OF INTEREST

The authors have no conflicts of interest to disclose.

REFERENCES

1. Alpert AB, Babbs G, Sanaeikia R, et al. Doing justice: ethical considerations identifying and researching transgender and gender diverse people in insurance claims data. *J Med Syst.* 2024;48(1):96. https://doi.org/10.1007/s10916-024-02111-w
2. Ganor O, Jolly D, Boskey ER. Nonsensical coding of gender-affirming procedures: a need for transgender-specific procedure codes. *J Am Coll Surg.* 2022;234(2):250–251. https://doi.org/10.1097/XCS.0000000000000015
3. Dai D, Charlton BM, Boskey ER, et al. Prevalence of gender-affirming surgical procedures among minors and adults in the US. *JAMA Netw Open.* 2024;7(6):e2418814. https://doi.org/10.1001/jamanetworkopen.2024.18814
4. Balkan E, Babbs G, Meyers DJ, et al. Gender-affirming surgery for transgender and gender diverse Medicare beneficiaries. *JAMA Netw Open.* 2025;8(5):e258072. https://doi.org/10.1001/jamanetworkopen.2025.8072
5. Baumgaertner E. Gender surgeries nearly tripled from 2016 through 2019, study finds. *New York Times.* August 23, 2023. Available at: https://www.nytimes.com/2023/08/23/health/transgender-surgery.html. Accessed October 23, 2025.
6. Wright JD, Chen L, Suzuki Y, Matsuo K, Hershman DL. National estimates of gender-affirming surgery in the US. *JAMA Netw Open.* 2023;6(8):e2330348. https://doi.org/10.1001/jamanetworkopen.2023.30348
7. Baker K, Restar A. Utilization and costs of gender-affirming care in a commercially insured transgender population. *J Law Med Ethics.* 2022;50(3):456–470. https://doi.org/10.1017/jme.2022.87

The Need to Focus on Flourishing LGBTQ+ Futures

B. Ethan Coston, PhD, and Stewart Landers, JD

ABOUT THE AUTHORS

B. Ethan Coston is an associate professor in the Department of Gender, Sexuality and Women's Studies, Virginia Commonwealth University, Richmond. Stewart Landers is associate editor emeritus for AJPH.

See also LGBTQ+ Well-Being and Joy, pp. 192–250.

In the field of mental health, well-being is something that is probably always top of mind. Indeed, many of us in the field rely on a range of approaches and tools to support our own efforts to do well. But even on our best days these tactics can fail us. When there is an seemingly endless supply of violence, trauma, grief, and pain in our worlds, flourishing mental health—or emotionally, psychologically, and socially feeling good and functioning well—may be even further out of reach.[1] So why do we offer a special section on LGBTQ+ (lesbian, gay, bisexual, transgender, queer, questioning, asexual, intersex, and other nonheterosexual, noncisgender) pride, joy, and flourishing? The current escalation of attacks on the LGBTQ+ community make this an important time to celebrate and understand the resilience and progress the community has made. Put simply: if not now, when?

EXPANDING THE SCOPE OF HEALTH RESEARCH

Scientists and scholars of LGBTQ+ health know that there is far more evidence on disparities, deficits, and diseases than on feeling good and functioning well. Some of this evidence is related to funding focus areas. For instance, in fiscal year 2024—before the various shifts in funding that happened internally—the National Institutes of Health RePORTER (Research Portfolio Online Reporting Tools: Expenditures and Results) showed that only 1.2% of all projects (and 2.1% of all money spent) focused on sexual and gender minority people, with nearly 80% falling under "prevention research" (i.e., studies that identify risk factors and evaluate interventions that reduce the risk of diseases or associated sequelae).

Research on transgender and gender-expansive people is not any more robust in its focus or analysis. In fact, not taking into account research specific to the so-called epidemiology of transgenderism or gender-affirming care (e.g., voice therapy, hormone use, and surgery), nearly 33% of all transgender health research produced from 1950 through 2016 focused on the "diagnosis and management of psychiatric comorbidities such as depression, anxiety, substance use, eating disorders, obsessive compulsive disorder, and autism in individuals with concurrent gender dysphoria,"[2(p123)] HIV risk and prevention (with a particular focus on transgender sex workers), and

HISTORY CORNER

7 YEARS AGO

50 Years After Stonewall . . . Empowerment, Expertise, and Energy

The Stonewall riots in June 1969 unleashed a torrent of gay activism, and the arena of lesbian, gay, bisexual, transgender, and queer or questioning (LGBTQ) health grew from a tiny seed into an essential aspect of the emerging queer communities. There is no escaping that the audacity of gays, lesbians, bisexuals, and drag queens (labeled as such at the time, but likely inclusive of people we call "transgender" today) who fought the police at the Stonewall lit a fire of empowerment among LGBTQ people across the United States and around the world. . . . The concept of LGBTQ health did not exist before Stonewall, and only began to emerge in the late '70s through the formation of the National Lesbian and Gay Health Foundation in 1977, which later became the National Lesbian and Gay Health Association. During this period, there was a growing body of work on the topic coming less from medicine than from queer political theory, psychology, social science, sociology, and education. . . . The underlying infrastructure to address the health issues of LGBTQ people continues to grow, fueled along the way by the Stonewall notions of empowerment and activism.

From *AJPH*, June 2019, pp. 849–850

AJPH February 2026, Vol. 116, No. 2

stigma, discrimination, and incarceration or criminalization.

PATHWAYS TO WELL-BEING

Although we recognize and acknowledge the importance of addressing the effects of disease burden, health risks, and care disparities, this special section is concerned primarily with activities, practices, research, education and curricula, policy briefs, programs, and community-led priority areas that highlight how resilience, thriving, flourishing, pride, and joy are also integral components of LGBTQ+ health and well-being. After all, health is not simply the absence of disease; it is also the ability to realize aspirations, satisfy needs, and adapt to or cope with the communal, social, and political environments around us.[3]

To do so successfully is complex, but research in this area shows promise for health promotion. For instance, integrating the measurement of flourishing into clinical care situates difficult treatment decisions within the broader context of what matters in a person's life, not merely how a treatment might affect them physically or mentally—an approach that exemplifies person-centered care.[4] What is more, reorienting health research, care, and policy toward achieving the goal of promoting human flourishing "can reinvigorate our thinking around health in a way that bends toward justice."[5(p100057)] Joy, whether directly or vicariously experienced, has been shown to foster positive communal relationships, strengthen connections to one's authentic self, and cultivate a sense of purpose or identity—offering insight into what could be achieved by integrating joy into mental health and well-being programs, initiatives, and interventions.[6]

A joy of life framework has shown particular promise in increasing elders' sense of belonging, participation in daily activities, feelings of being valuable and useful, and small glimmers of well-being.[7] Finally, recent work seeking to balance deficit-focused research on psychological stressors has found support for minority strengths models that link positive health behaviors and mental health to identity pride, self-esteem, and resilience—factors bolstered by a range of strengths processes, including social support, community consciousness, self-compassion, hope, authenticity, and relationship intimacy.[8,9]

These are just some of the ways that resilience, flourishing, pride, and joy positively affect health, which this special section expands on. Adrian et al. (p. 214) examine "sex-positive, strengths-based prevention materials designed by LGBT-led AIDS service organizations (ASOs) in the first decade of the HIV/AIDS epidemic." To understand the historical record of sex-positive HIV prevention messaging, they focus primarily on the work of the Gay Men's Health Crisis in its first decade of existence to draw on new collections of archival material and oral histories, as well as their own extensive interviews with Gay Men's Health Crisis alumni. The authors highlight three themes: gay liberation, community connectedness, and eroticism. An early Gay Men's Health Crisis workshop had the objective of developing "skills for building compassionate, altruistic relationships that extended beyond casual sex."

Rhodes (p. 202), commenting on the article by Adrian et al., notes that their work with Latine immigrant communities and queer people in rural Appalachia builds on "their realities—who they are and what they value—not simply

HISTORY CORNER

25 YEARS AGO

Why Lesbian, Gay, Bisexual, and Transgender Public Health?

Despite the many differences that separate them, LGBT people share remarkably similar experiences related to stigma, discrimination, rejection, and violence across cultures and locales. In the United States, gay men and lesbians are subject to legal discrimination in housing, employment, and basic civil rights. Sodomy laws, which brand gays and lesbians as criminals in 16 states, are often the basis for harassment and discrimination. Transgender individuals are stigmatized, discriminated against, and ridiculed in encounters with even those entrusted with their care. LGBT people fare better in some areas (e.g., parts of the European Community) than in others, but they are still subject to persecution and discrimination in many regions of the world. LGBT people have formed communities that bridge their many differences. These communities have provided safe spaces, developed norms and values, and created institutions where LGBT identities and relationships can be acknowledged and respected.

From *AJPH*, June 2001, p. 856

their sexual risks." He finds Adrean et al. to be asserting that research can go beyond disease prevention to create "space for LGBTQ+ people to feel valued, understood, and connected." Rhodes further calls on researchers to expand our knowledge of "how cultural context and grassroots expertise inform successful interventions and programs," which should resonate with public health practitioners and policymakers as well.

Schall et al. (p. 192) explore the directive from the current US presidential administration to the National Institutes of Health that terminated most, if not all, research on transgender health and redirected future research toward the study of transition regret, detransitioning, and transgender health services as a form of "body mutilation" rather than necessary and affirming care. Reflecting on the ethical principles of beneficence and autonomy, they reassert the reality that the great majority of transgender people find satisfaction, happiness, and increased wellness following gender-affirming care. This care may include help with vocal expression or hair removal or may be surgical procedures for which postsurgical regret levels are extremely low (a large majority of such transgender care has lower regret levels than other forms of surgical intervention). Their findings show how transgender health care and services necessarily support transgender people in living their fullest lives.

Similarly, Gaedecke et al. (p. 205) report qualitative findings from a longitudinal mixed-methods cohort study in which transgender and gender-diverse adults describe the benefits of gender-affirming surgery. With insights into how surgical intervention brought relief and ease, confidence, and a new sense of access to experience the world in ways they never thought possible, this work draws attention to how feeling connected to and positive about one's own body can open up possibilities for deeper and more meaningful social connection and self-improvement.

Furthermore, in a Notes From The Field article that focuses on the benefits of supporting social transition–related care, Mackenzie et al. (p. 210) describe a transgender youth–driven school–community organizing process that led to concrete institutional (e.g., all gender bathroom access was increased) and policy shifts. The goal of this initiative was to "identify opportunities for environmental change to support transgender and nonbinary student health and well-being." The model is a blueprint to empower other interventions of its kind to build school environments that support the health and well-being of all transgender students.

Ogunbajo et al. (p. 229) look at how gender affirmation, especially legal recognition and access to gender-affirming health care, is associated with interest in adoption among a cohort of transgender and nonbinary people in Washington State. Among participants whose gender goals included legal gender affirmation, the researchers quantified the number of legal documents participants had updated (e.g., passports, driver's licenses or state identification cards, social security cards, birth certificates). They found that updating one or more of these documents to one's current gender or name was more common among respondents interested in adoption.

Legal and structural affirmation are also highlighted in the work of Agor et al. (p. 222), which examines the resilience processes of sexual and gender-diverse

HISTORY CORNER

25 YEARS AGO

Uneasy Promises: Sexuality, Health, and Human Rights

Recent global work to develop the concepts of health and human rights includes at least 3 different approaches. One of the first evolved from an examination of the causal links between human rights abuses and health. This approach can encompass the connection between torture because of sexual orientation and its health effects. A second approach searches for the human rights effects of public health practices, such as discriminatory and coercive strategies concerning HIV testing. The third, more comprehensive approach examines the potential synergistic effects between health and human rights; it postulates that "promoting and protecting health requires explicit and concrete efforts to promote and protect human rights and dignity." This approach could take on the many complicated ways that discrimination on the basis of sex, race, sexual orientation, HIV status, age, or disability, for example, affects health status. It could include scrutiny into how intersecting discriminations, as in sexualized forms of race discrimination, affect health, or the right to health. . . . [O]ne strength of human rights work is that it meshes formal treaty doctrines with grassroots activism and critiques of power, 'the legitimate territory of those who make political demands about basic justice.'

From *AJPH*, June 2001, pp. 861–862.

survival migrants. Examining the sophisticated identity management strategies they employ in high-structural stigma environments and recognizing the paradox that resilience is both powerful and burdensome, they highlight "how sexual and gender-diverse survival migrants use individual strengths and multilevel assets to progress from immediate survival to long-term flourishing" in the United States. They end with recommendations for public health practice (e.g., trauma-informed peer support groups) as well as policy reform suggestions relative to current asylum processes.

Finally, Mackenzie et al. (p. 210) reaffirm the centrality of family, broadly defined to include chosen family, to the queer community. Children raised in LGBTQ+ families do not differ in health, family relationships, or adult outcomes from those raised by cisgender, heterosexual parents. Therefore, policies that support child-rearing—such as supports for pregnant people and newborn children, HeadStart, and antipoverty programs that assist with housing and address food insecurity—must define family broadly enough to include queer families.

BUILDING CONDITIONS FOR FLOURISHING

As the contributions to this special section show, human life is complex. Risk and resilience, sorrow and joy, and stigma and pride can coexist in people's lived experiences. To attend to these complexities, it is essential that we continue to cultivate research in asset-focused areas, using strengths-based frameworks. We cannot simply triage health issues, attending narrowly to singular diseases, diagnoses, or outcomes. This fragmented approach will never fully meet the complex health needs of our communities, nor will it adequately address some of the root causes of those needs.[10] Instead, we should be "providing the tools and resources that individuals and communities need for facing today's challenges before they develop downstream consequences."[11] Ultimately, we hope that this special section—with its specific focus on LGBTQ+ people—encourages individuals, practitioners, clinicians, policymakers, and communities to develop ways of living and healing that promote meaning, resilience, and well-being across the life course.[12] AJPH

CORRESPONDENCE

Correspondence should be sent to B. Ethan Coston, 919 W. Franklin St, Richmond, VA 23284 (e-mail: bmcoston@vcu.edu). Reprints can be ordered at https://www.ajph.org by clicking the "Reprints" link.

PUBLICATION INFORMATION

Full Citation: Coston BE, Landers S. The need to focus on flourishing LGBTQ+ futures. *Am J Public Health*. 2026;116(2):188–191.

Acceptance Date: November 15, 2025.

DOI: https://doi.org/10.2105/AJPH.2025.308364

ORCID iDs:

B. Ethan Coston https://orcid.org/0000-0002-6511-4362

Stewart Landers https://orcid.org/0009-0005-5101-4108

CONTRIBUTORS

The authors contributed equally to this article.

CONFLICTS OF INTEREST

The authors have no conflicts of interest to report.

REFERENCES

1. Keyes CLM. The mental health continuum: from languishing to flourishing in life. *J Health Soc Behav*. 2002;43(2):207–222.
2. Wanta JW, Unger CA. Review of the transgender literature: where do we go from here. *Transgend Health*. 2017;2(1):119–128. https://doi.org/10.1089/trgh.2017.0004
3. Kickbusch I. Health promotion: a global perspective. *Can J Public Health*. 1986;77(5):321–326.
4. VanderWeele TJ, McNeely E, Koh HK. Reimagining health—flourishing. *JAMA*. 2019;321(17):1667–1668. https://doi.org/10.1001/jama.2019.3035
5. Willen SS, Williamson AF, Walsh CC, Hyman M, Tootle W. Rethinking flourishing: critical insights and qualitative perspectives from the US Midwest. *SSM Ment Health*. 2022;2:100057. https://doi.org/10.1016/j.ssmmh.2021.100057
6. Roberts M, Appiah R. The complexities of joy: a qualitative study of joy cultivation, loss of joy, and happiness in British adults. *Int J Qual Stud Health Well-being*. 2025;20(1):2508946. https://doi.org/10.1080/17482631.2025.2508946
7. Rinnan E, André B, Drageset J, Garåsen H, Espnes GA, Haugan G. Joy of life in nursing homes: a qualitative study of what constitutes the essence of joy of life in elderly individuals living in Norwegian nursing homes. *Scand J Caring Sci*. 2018;32(4):1468–1476. https://doi.org/10.1111/scs.12598
8. Perrin PB, Sutter ME, Trujillo MA, Henry RS, Pugh Jr M. The minority strengths model: development and initial path analytic validation in racially/ethnically diverse LGBTQ individuals. *J Clin Psychol*. 2020;76(1):118–136. https://doi.org/10.1002/jclp.22850
9. Parmenter JG, Winter SD, Clements ZA, Alexander K, Taylor H. How community and individual strengths "fill our cup": a preliminary strengths-based psychological mediation framework for LGBTQIA+ communities. *J Couns Psychol*. 2025;72(5):614–626. https://doi.org/10.1037/cou0000807
10. Lynch J. *A Whole Person Approach to Wellbeing: Building Sense of Safety*. New York, NY: Routledge; 2022.
11. Witt CM, Chiaramonte D, Berman S, et al. Defining health in a comprehensive context: a new definition of integrative health. *Am J Prev Med*. 2017;53(1):134–137. https://doi.org/10.1016/j.amepre.2016.11.029
12. The time is now for a whole-person health approach to public health. *Public Health Rep*. 2023;138(4):561–564. https://doi.org/10.1177/00333549231154583

Dangers of a Politically Motivated Research Agenda on Transgender Health

Theodore E. Schall, PhD, MSW, MBE, Jacob D. Moses, PhD, Elizabeth A. Dietz, PhD, Laura E. Stamm, PhD, Justin Penny, DO, MA, and Ayden I. Scheim, PhD

ABOUT THE AUTHORS

Theodore E. Schall is with the School of Public Health and Health Sciences, University of Massachusetts Amherst. Jacob D. Moses is with the School of Public and Population Health, University of Texas Medical Branch, Galveston. Elizabeth A. Dietz is with the Center for Biology and Society, Arizona State University, Tempe. Laura E. Stamm is with the Department of Medicine, University of Rochester Medical Center, Rochester, NY. Justin Penny is with Allina Health, Minneapolis, MN. Ayden I. Scheim is with the Dornsife School of Public Health, Drexel University, Philadelphia, PA.

See also LGBTQ+ Well-Being and Joy, pp. 188–250.

On April 3, 2025, *Nature News* revealed that the current administration had directed the National Institutes of Health (NIH) to study "regret and detransition" among transgender and gender-diverse (TGD) children and adults.[1] The directive echoed the language of "chemical and surgical mutilation" used in recent executive orders. It was noteworthy for including social transition (e.g., adoption of a gender-concordant name, pronouns, gender expression, or gender role[2]) and encompassing both adult and pediatric medical care. Simultaneously, the administration terminated more than $800 million in funding for lesbian, gay, bisexual, transgender, and queer (LGBTQ+) health studies because "research programs based on gender identity are often unscientific, have little identifiable return on investment, and do nothing to enhance the health of many Americans."[3]

The NIH directive is just one among many recent attacks on transgender rights in service of an ideological goal that has been described by some proponents as "eradicating transgenderism."[4] Research funding is being weaponized through both cancellation of existing grants and mobilization of federal agencies to target vulnerable populations. These actions discount existing evidence supporting the careful provision of gender-affirming care and instead call for biased studies that demonstrate the risk of "detransition" (a term out of favor with transgender communities), the likelihood of regret, and the presumed harms associated with both.

Here we identify and critique three assumptions embedded in the federal funding directive that will undercut the rigor of any results produced under it. The first assumption is that gender-affirming care is mutilation, a form of violence rather than medical care. The second is that the presence of regret in any form is sufficient to discredit the legitimacy or legality of a medical practice. The third assumption is that gaps in high-quality evidence stem from the illegitimacy of transgender medicine rather than the history and politics of research in the field. We address each assumption to argue that this directive will undermine the evidence base, with foreseeable negative consequences for researchers and patients alike.

MUTILATION

Characterizing gender-affirming care as "chemical and surgical mutilation" is not a neutral or scientific description but rather a statement about this administration's position regarding the legitimacy of gender-affirming care. This characterization implicitly denies the systemic drivers of TGD health disparities and locates the suffering of TGD people in care itself. In effect, the NIH has been charged with concluding that gender-affirming care is harmful before the research to prove it has even been performed.

By contrast, most TGD people experience gender-affirming care as essential physical and mental health care.[5] The term "mutilation" discredits the health care professionals who provide gender-affirming care by suggesting that they are at best mistaken about helping TGD people thrive[6] and at worst knowingly harming their patients. Furthermore, the inappropriate conflation of gender-affirming care with iatrogenic harm sets up a predictable, tragic next policy move: a national ban on gender-affirming care for TGD people of all ages. Such a move would wrest authority over what constitutes ethical care away from every major medical association, which all hold gender-affirming care to be medically necessary, and redefine a private

AJPH February 2026, Vol. 116, No. 2

medical concern as a matter of public interest.

REGRET AND "DETRANSITION"

The NIH directive's focus on regret parallels ongoing arguments over the implications of regret in abortion care.[7] As in abortion debates, critics of gender-affirming care suggest that the mere possibility of regret merits categorical prohibition and calls for studies on the presumed harms of later-regretted transitions. Conversely, defenders of gender-affirming care have cited low rates of regret to substantiate its effectiveness. In pointing out that two sides of an increasingly polarized debate have invoked regret, we do not intend to suggest that gender-affirming care lacks sufficient evidence, nor do we equate the merits of these approaches. Our intention is to point out that, as is true in most health policy debates, the dichotomous approaches here reflect diverging underlying values. A public health approach to TGD care is typically aligned with the ethical principles of beneficence and autonomy.

Studies show that almost all TGD people feel better after receiving gender-affirming care. Although post-surgical regret is a common phenomenon after many types of surgery, the reported prevalence of regret after gender-affirming surgery is remarkably low, ranging from 0.3% to 1.0%, as compared with much higher rates for common surgeries such as breast augmentation (5%–9%) and bariatric surgery (19.5%).[8] Similarly, less than 1% of US adults surveyed in the largest national TGD survey to date who were receiving hormones reported being "a little" or "a lot less satisfied" with their lives, whereas the vast majority reported improvements in satisfaction.[9]

Critics and proponents agree that the research base for pediatric gender-affirming care is less robust than that for adults, yet recent studies of youths have consistently revealed high rates of satisfaction and low rates of regret. A systematic review of youth social transition showed that when adolescents were protected from harassment at school, social transition was not associated with negative long-term mental health effects.[2] Similarly, an analysis of 2023 survey data showed a 97% continuation rate among adolescents prescribed puberty blockers or hormones, with just 4% expressing any form of regret.[10]

There is no consensus about how to operationalize the concepts of regret and "detransition." Nevertheless, narrowly defined studies that treat detransition as a binary variable are fundamentally out of step with what is known by those with lived experience and professional expertise about transition. TGD people may pause, stop, or restart medical treatment in response to shifts in or accomplishment of embodiment goals, reproductive desires, social pressure, access to care, or medical contraindications. Moreover, it is problematic to attribute labels of regret and detransition to a person on the basis of a specific pattern in health administrative data, such as the discontinuation of hormones. Defining these terms as failures of medical care or evidence of care having been offered inappropriately fails to encompass the complexity of patient decisions.

It is, however, possible to rigorously study regret and its social contexts as a growing body of literature already suggests. What we know about "detransition" is that many people pursue it not because of a fundamental change in their understanding of themselves but because of external pressures such as societal stigma and family rejection.[11] Those researching detransition call for better care, not less care.[12] What we learn about the experiences of people who regret having received gender-affirming care should be used to improve how care is delivered and patients are supported in their decision making. It should not serve as a pretext to prohibit others from obtaining medically necessary care.

EVIDENCE AND EPISTEMIC MARGINALIZATION

In clear opposition to the NIH directive, there is a strong consensus about the medical necessity of gender-affirming care among researchers and providers.[13] Some proponents have suggested that evidence alone proves that such care is legitimate and appropriate. Yet, as the national backlash against access to gender-affirming care has shown, evidence without context and interpretation cannot dictate health policy or resolve conflicts regarding underlying values.[14]

As the evidence for affirming transgender people's gender identities has grown in recent years, so too have objections about the absence of certain kinds of evidence, namely randomized controlled trials (RCTs). Critics contend that the evidence base is "low quality" because standards for systematic review of evidence generally privilege randomized controlled trials and discount the observational studies that form much of the evidence base for TGD medicine. Given the strong, consistent evidence supporting the benefits of gender-affirming care, researchers are not in a state of uncertainty about the comparative merits of standards of care and placebos (clinical equipoise[15]); as such, study designs that randomize TGD patients to a nontreatment control group are generally ethically unacceptable.[16] Fortunately, observational studies can offer robust, ethical data without the harm of preventing access to treatments with known benefits.

TGD medicine is not unique in having a contested evidence base: making medical judgments with limited or emerging forms of evidence is standard in many specialties, particularly in pediatrics.[17] Yet TGD medicine is different from many other specialties inasmuch as the absence of sufficient quality evidence reflects historical epistemic marginalization, defined as the systematic exclusion of certain groups or voices from the creation of knowledge. Excluding marginalized populations from the production of scientific knowledge informing their care undermines the quality of knowledge and ultimately patient-centered care.

Mainstream medical and political actors have long marginalized the provision of TGD care and the production of research on transgender health.[18] One violent example was the 1933 Nazi burning of Magnus Hirschfeld's Institute of Sexology, which pioneered research on transsexuality.[19] In the United States, the 1980s saw politicized closure of gender clinics at academic medical centers, which stunted the growing field of transgender health research.[20] These institutional shifts drove much of this work into private clinics that lacked research infrastructure and incentives for providers to publish.[20] The fragmented US health care system has also made health service research with small populations relatively onerous to conduct, which is why the most robust data about gender-related care come from countries with integrated health systems.[21]

Both supporters and opponents of gender-affirming care note gaps in the US evidence base, although they disagree about their causes and nature. Opponents argue that negative outcomes such as regret have been systematically excluded from study. Yet, regret has been studied since the establishment of standards for gender-affirming care in 1979.[22] Then and now, antitransgender policies have epistemically marginalized both TGD communities and TGD health researchers. Efforts to study authentic transgender experiences—especially patient well-being—have been stymied by lack of funding, publisher reluctance, the relative paucity of transgender researchers in academic roles, and legislative bans on gender-affirming care. Thus, there are well-known gaps in the evidence base for gender-affirming care surrounding long-term hormone use and surgical outcomes, health throughout the TGD life span, and sexual and reproductive health.[23]

The trend over the past decade had been toward federal prioritization of more rigorous research on transgender health. For example, in 2015 the NIH established the Sexual and Gender Minority Research Office, which in 2023 implemented the Expanding the Evidence Base in Gender-Affirming Care initiative to develop a consensus on research priorities in this field. Major institutions such as the National Cancer Institute began recommending the collection of gender identity data across treatment and research contexts. The NIH directive arrived in the context of a reversal of this trend: within the first three months of the current administration's term, the Sexual and Gender Minority Research Office was disbanded.

Transgender marginalization extends well beyond epistemic matters, into most domains of well-being. TGD people are disproportionately vulnerable to violence, discrimination, unemployment, homelessness, food insecurity, and lack of medical care.[24] We know this because of community-led research efforts (such as the US Transgender Survey) and a body of increasingly robust research on TGD health. A research agenda skewed toward the negative consequences of gender-affirming care will omit, and perhaps outright deny, these structural barriers to well-being. These are the central—and often enormous—problems in TGD people's lives, and they risk being officially ignored.

IMPLICATIONS FOR RESEARCHERS

This NIH directive should be understood as a hijacking of the health research enterprise in service of an oppressive ideology. It serves an unscientific worldview in which human sex is a strict binary that is inextricable from gender. Antitransgender advocates are explicit about wanting to exclude TGD people from public life and ban gender-affirming care. Mobilization of the NIH and researchers to create the evidence to support these oppressive policies poses foreseeable harms for both TGD and cisgender people.

Framing personal choices about expression as a federal research priority is especially concerning. The directive's inclusion of social transition reflects the administration's commitment to enforcing binary gender expression well beyond health care. When gender is rigidly defined for LGBTQ+ people, it is also easier to rigidly define it for all.

As with restrictions around reproductive care access, restrictions around gender expression limit bodily autonomy and the right to self-determination. Recent state "bathroom ban" laws evoke an earlier wave of cross-dressing bans that proliferated in the second half of the 19th century and targeted transgender, queer, and intersex people, along with cisgender women who did not conform to contemporary standards of femininity.[25] These policies excluded LGBTQ+ people and women from public spaces such as the workforce and made society less free and less equitable.

Scientists should not be complicit with this dangerous directive or the ideology it represents. With many TGD health researchers facing the loss of their scientific careers, it is unclear who will be left to conduct rigorous research on gender-affirming care. Experienced TGD health researchers (particularly those who are TGD themselves) may be systematically excluded from leading NIH grants because of new application screening standards. Although any new source of funding may be appealing in this context, we encourage our colleagues to carefully consider whether it is possible to conduct ethical research under the banner of an institution that intends to further epistemically marginalize transgender people. Scientifically valuable research can be conducted on topics of regret and detransition, but the directive's framing of these issues is at odds with the expert consensus. Researchers should seek admittedly limited funding sources outside the federal government so that they can maintain the academic freedom and objectivity necessary to produce high-quality evidence about the full range of outcomes—including satisfaction and regret—in all of their complex dimensions.

CONCLUSION

Public health has recognized the health disparities faced by the TGD population; until recently, this fact was reflected by the inclusion of TGD people in a range of Healthy People 2030 goals. If provision of adult gender-affirming care is halted because of biased "evidence" of its harms, the human cost will be widespread suffering and death. Not all transgender people experience gender dysphoria, but for those who do, the experience is by definition profoundly distressing and worthy of medical attention. It is not ethical to simply ignore known medical needs in service of a political agenda. Now more than ever, high-quality research, driven by investigator expertise and TGD community values, is needed on the full spectrum of outcomes of gender-affirming care.

Private funders and sanctuary states have important roles to play in ensuring that rigorous TGD health research continues to be funded, even though this research likely cannot proceed at the same scale that would have been possible with federal funding. Whether or not they can find alternative funding sources, public health researchers have a vital role to play in not manufacturing ideologically motivated evidence that will further harm the health of a vulnerable population. AJPH

CORRESPONDENCE

Correspondence should be sent to Theodore E. Schall, PhD, MSW, MBE, Room 325 Arnold House, 715 North Pleasant St, Amherst, MA 01003 (e-mail: tschall@umass.edu). Reprints can be ordered at https://www.ajph.org by clicking the "Reprints" link.

PUBLICATION INFORMATION

Full Citation: Schall TE, Moses JD, Dietz EA, Stamm LE, Penny J, Scheim AI. Dangers of a politically motivated research agenda on transgender health. *Am J Public Health*. 2026;116(2):192–196.

Acceptance Date: September 9, 2025.

DOI: https://doi.org/10.2105/AJPH.2025.308288

ORCID iDs:

Theodore E. Schall https://orcid.org/0000-0002-0353-2657

Jacob D. Moses https://orcid.org/0000-0001-8089-3870

Laura E. Stamm https://orcid.org/0009-0003-4865-2972

Justin Penny https://orcid.org/0000-0003-1385-9570

Ayden I. Scheim https://orcid.org/0000-0001-8498-9829

CONTRIBUTORS

T. E. Schall conceptualized the article and prepared the original draft. J. D. Moses, J. Penny, E. A. Dietz, L. E. Stamm, and A. I. Scheim participated in revising the article for important intellectual content.

ACKNOWLEDGMENTS

We thank Christene DeJong for her assistance in preparing the article.

Note. The views of the authors do not necessarily represent the views of their institutions or funders.

CONFLICTS OF INTEREST

The authors have no potential or actual conflicts of interest to disclose.

REFERENCES

1. Kozlov M. Exclusive: Trump White House directs NIH to study regret after transgender people transition. Available at: https://www.nature.com/articles/d41586-025-01029-8. Accessed September 6, 2025.
2. Turban JL, King D, Li JJ, Keuroghlian AS. Timing of social transition for transgender and gender diverse youth, K-12 harassment, and adult mental health outcomes. *J Adolesc Health*. 2021;69(6):991–998. https://doi.org/10.1016/j.jadohealth.2021.06.001
3. Chen A. NIH terminates ongoing grants for LGBTQ+ research. Available at: https://www.statnews.com/2025/03/03/nih-terminates-ongoing-grants-for-lgbtq-research. Accessed September 6, 2025.
4. Gambino L. Anti-trans rhetoric took center stage at CPAC amid hostile Republican efforts. Available at: https://www.theguardian.com/us-news/2023/mar/07/cpac-anti-trans-rhetoric. Accessed September 6, 2025.

5. Restar AJ. Gender-affirming care is preventative care. *Lancet Reg Health Am.* 2023;24:100544. https://doi.org/10.1016/j.lana.2023.100544
6. Shirin A, Daniello M, Stamm L. Providers' beliefs and values: understanding their approach to gender-affirming care. *J Prim Care Community Health.* 2025;16:21501319241312574. https://doi.org/10.1177/21501319241312574
7. Watson K. A piece of my mind. Reframing regret. *JAMA.* 2014;311(1):27–29. https://doi.org/10.1001/jama.2013.283739
8. Thornton SM, Edalatpour A, Gast KM. A systematic review of patient regret after surgery—a common phenomenon in many specialties but rare within gender-affirmation surgery. *Am J Surg.* 2024;234:68–73. https://doi.org/10.1016/j.amjsurg.2024.04.021
9. Rastogi A, Menard L, Miller GH, et al. Health and wellbeing: a report of the 2022 US Transgender Survey. Available at: https://ustranssurvey.org/download-reports. Accessed September 6, 2025.
10. Olson KR, Raber G, Gallagher NM. Levels of satisfaction and regret with gender-affirming medical care in adolescence. *JAMA Pediatr.* 2024;178(12):1354–1361. https://doi.org/10.1001/jamapediatrics.2024.4527
11. Roberts CM, Klein DA, Adirim TA, Schvey NA, Hisle-Gorman E. Continuation of gender-affirming hormones among transgender adolescents and adults. *J Clin Endocrinol Metab.* 2022;107(9):e3937–e3943. https://doi.org/10.1210/clinem/dgac251
12. Maragos AC, Brown C, Allen LR. Lived experiences: exploring detransition narratives. *Int J Transgend Health.* 2025;26(1):215–234. https://doi.org/10.1080/26895269.2025.2458696
13. Coleman E, Radix AE, Bouman WP, et al. Standards of care for the health of transgender and gender diverse people, version 8. *Int J Transgend Health.* 2022;23(suppl 1):S1–S259. https://doi.org/10.1080/26895269.2022.2100644
14. Fausto-Sterling A. Science won't settle trans rights. Available at: https://www.bostonreview.net/articles/anne-fausto-sterling-who-speaks-science. Accessed September 6, 2025.
15. Freedman B. Equipoise and the ethics of clinical research. *N Engl J Med.* 1987;317(3):141–145. https://doi.org/10.1056/nejm198707163170304
16. Ashley F, Tordoff DM, Olson-Kennedy J, Restar AJ. Randomized-controlled trials are methodologically inappropriate in adolescent transgender healthcare. *Int J Transgend Health.* 2024;25(3):407–418. https://doi.org/10.1080/26895269.2023.2218357
17. Howick J, Koletsi D, Pandis N, et al. The quality of evidence for medical interventions does not improve or worsen: a metaepidemiological study of Cochrane reviews. *J Clin Epidemiol.* 2020;126:154–159. https://doi.org/10.1016/j.jclinepi.2020.08.005
18. Coulter RWS, Kenst KS, Bowen, DJ, Scout. Research funded by the National Institutes of Health on the health of lesbian, gay, bisexual, and transgender populations. *Am J Public Health.* 2014;104(2):e105–e112. https://doi.org/10.2105/AJPH.2013.301501
19. Li A. *Wondrous Transformations: A Maverick Physician, the Science of Hormones, and the Birth of the Transgender Revolution.* UNC Press Books; 2023.
20. Magrath WJ. The fall of the nation's first gender-affirming surgery clinic. *Ann Intern Med.* 2022;175(10):1462–1467. https://doi.org/10.7326/m22-1480
21. Slagstad K. Bureaucratizing medicine: creating a gender identity clinic in the welfare state. *Isis.* 2022;113(3):469–490. https://doi.org/10.1086/721140
22. Edgerton MT, Knorr NJ, Callison JR. The surgical treatment of transsexual patients: limitations and indications. *Plast Reconstr Surg.* 1970;45(1):38–46. https://doi.org/10.1097/00006534-197001000-00006
23. Veale JF, Deutsch MB, Devor AH, et al. Setting a research agenda in trans health: an expert assessment of priorities and issues by trans and nonbinary researchers. *Int J Transgend Health.* 2022;23(4):392–408. https://doi.org/10.1080/26895269.2022.2044425
24. National Academies of Sciences, Engineering, and Medicine. Understanding the well-being of LGBTQI+ populations. Available at: https://nap.nationalacademies.org/read/25877/chapter/1#xii. Accessed September 6, 2025.
25. Redburn K. Before equal protection: the fall of cross-dressing bans and the transgender legal movement, 1963–86. *Law Hist Rev.* 2022;40(4):679–723. https://doi.org/10.1017/S0738248022000384

Flourishing Families: Promoting Public Health and Reproductive Justice for All by Protecting and Supporting LGBTQ+ Families in Policy and Practice

Sonja Mackenzie, DrPH, ScM, Nesta N. Johnson, JD, Joanna E. Scheib, PhD, Liam Kali, LM, and Jordan Wilson, BA

ABOUT THE AUTHORS

Sonja Mackenzie is with the Department of Public Health, Santa Clara University, Santa Clara, CA. Nesta N. Johnson is a Family Liberation Attorney in Ashley, PA. Joanna E. Scheib is with the Department of Psychology, University of California, Davis, and The Sperm Bank of California in Berkeley. Liam Kali is with Maia Midwifery and Fertility Services in Seattle, WA. Jordan Wilson is with COLAGE (Children of Lesbians and Gays Everywhere) in Providence, RI.

See also LGBTQ+ Well-Being and Joy, pp. 188–250.

We are researchers, practitioners, and advocates working with and for LGBTQ+ people (lesbian, gay, bisexual, transgender, queer or questioning, or people whose identities are outside dominant groups of heterosexual sexual identities). We observe with alarm the medical and scientific establishment's muted responses to the onslaught of executive orders narrowly targeting LGBTQ+ people and broadly endangering reproductive health and autonomy. Efforts to relegate sexual and gender minorities to invisible, second-class status are the opening salvo in a broader attack upon the rights, autonomy, and dignity of women; racial, ethnic, and religious minorities; immigrants; and people with disabilities.

The current assault on the reproductive rights and medical autonomy of women and LGBTQ+ people is ironically cloaked under the guise of promoting their well-being. Orders intended to end legal recognition of transgender and nonbinary people (e.g., limiting access to identity documents, health care, services, and facilities); permitting discrimination on the basis of sexual orientation, gender identity, and gender expression (SOGIE); halting foreign medical aid; and reinstating the abortion "gag rule" abroad are clearly harmful.[1] Perhaps less apparent are the pernicious motives underlying plans to improve access to in vitro fertilization (IVF) for "loving and longing mothers and fathers."[2] All evidence indicates that such policies will deliberately exclude hopeful parents who are LGBTQ+ or otherwise deemed unfit to produce "beautiful" babies.[2] The aim: to selectively promote the reproduction of people with traits deemed "desirable" while hindering the reproduction of people with so-called "undesirable" traits.

Such reproductive governance will codify discrimination, entrench existing inequities, and, coupled with outdated parentage laws, leave many LGBTQ+ or queer parents and their children legally vulnerable ("LGBTQ+" and "queer" are used interchangeably herein). An especially insidious aspect of this regressive reproductive crusade is its effort to (re)define the concept of family and to weaponize the nuclear family—described as "the greatest form of governance known to humankind"[3]—as a primary vehicle of social and economic oppression. US law derives from English common law, in which the family as a legal structure existed to secure patrilineal inheritance, yielding the "presumption of legitimacy" for marital children. Under "coverture," aspects of which existed in the United States until the 1970s, married women had no autonomous legal existence. The nuclear family enables capitalism by privatizing and devaluing caregiving labor, thereby disadvantaging many women as wage arners. The campaign to define family narrowly as heterosexual, cisgender, dyadic, and procreative pathologizes and disadvantages childless, childfree, single-parent, multiparent, extended, chosen, and Tribal families. Moreover, this narrow family model excludes the vast majority of US families, which are diverse and flexible in structure.[4]

As researchers and medical, health, and legal professionals specializing in LGBTQ+ reproduction, parenting, and families, we have witnessed firsthand the struggle for recognition and against oppression, the fostering of resiliency, and the cultivation of well-being, pride,

AJPH February 2026, Vol. 116, No. 2

and joy within LGBTQ+ families. We have studied reproductive technologies from donor insemination[5] to the stratifications of assisted reproduction (including gamete donation and IVF).[6,7] We have advised on US policy relating to family, reproduction, and health care[8] and witnessed the heartbreak of genetically unrelated parents denied access to children they parented since birth.[9] We have worked with thousands of people raised by LGBTQ+ parents, who are directly experiencing the harmful impact of anti-LGBTQ+ policy and rhetoric and increasingly fear for their families' safety. We have assisted tens of thousands of LGBTQ+ people through planning, conceiving, gestating, and birthing babies into loving families.[10] "Pride" as celebrated by racial and sexual minority communities denotes "a collective sense of self-worth," while "joy"—contra fleeting "happiness"—signifies "the ability to affirm the goodness of life even in the midst of sorrow."[11,12] Evocatively, children often are described as their families' "pride and joy."

From the depth of our expertise, we wish to signal a reminder, a warning, and a call to action for all whose mandate is to promote public health and well-being.

FIRST, THE REMINDER

The concept of family is integral to the queer community, and children raised by LGBTQ+ parents and same-sex couples fare similarly to children raised by cisgender, heterosexual-couple parents.

Family Is Central to LGBTQ+ Communities

Family—which we define broadly as relationships of care over time that may or may not involve genetic ties, sexual intimacy, reproduction, or child-rearing and may include individuals of varying ages within or across generations—has always been a central structure supporting queer well-being throughout history, whether recognized or not.[13] LGBTQ+ people embrace family so fundamentally as to claim the Sister Sledge song, "We Are Family" as a cultural anthem. LGBTQ+ families are often referred to as "chosen families," evoking the ways in which LGBTQ+ communities create families, which transcend heteronormative, biologically based family structures.[14]

Narrow conceptions of family result in concrete harms in the context of federal policies. In a 2020 report, The Center for American Progress urged federal policymakers to understand that the failure to "fully recognize that chosen families exist causes real harm . . . from the insult of not being recognized to not being included in or covered by certain benefits or programs."[15] Defining family informs a wide range of policies and practices, including determining access to employment benefits, custodial rights, survivorship benefits, housing access, and more. Many LGBTQ+ families include children: currently, nearly one in five US LGBTQ+ adults (18%) are parenting children younger than 18 years—a total of 2.6 million families. Because Black LGBTQ+ adults are more likely than White adults to be parenting (23% vs 17%), and LGBTQ+ parents are more likely to experience poverty (33%) than LGBTQ+ nonparents (21%), policies impacting LGBTQ+ parents and their children disproportionately impact families of color and poor families.[16] Queer families promote lifelong well-being, providing a crucial source of support and means of survival amid pervasive homophobia and transphobia and rejection and abuse inflicted by families of origin.[17] Our professional and personal experiences of queer family inform our recognition of the importance of defining "family" broadly to include nongenetic kinship and diverse family structures.

The Kids Are Alright

The data are crystal clear: the quality and security of familial relationships matter for children's well-being; the gender or sexual orientation of their parent(s) does not. Regardless of how measured—whether in population-based samples or among subsets of families, such as those created through assisted reproduction—children raised by LGBTQ+ parents and same-sex couples fare similarly to children raised by cisgender, heterosexual-couple parents in health, quality of family relationships, and outcomes in adulthood.[18] Queer people build families in diverse ways, parenting children born through assisted reproduction, adopted privately or from foster care, and originated during previous different-sex relationships, within a variety of family structures. These kids are alright. Indeed, LGBTQ+ families and the providers who serve them are "ahead of the curve" in some respects. Surviving eras of invisibility and forced "passing," criminalization, and violence has led queer families to value trust, honesty, and intentionality.

The benefits of these qualities, especially honesty, in LGBTQ+ families support donor-conceived person advocates' call for early disclosure of donor-assisted reproduction. The Sperm Bank of California—a nonprofit originally created to serve lesbian couples and single women being refused care elsewhere—has always supported parents sharing "donor origin stories" with children and created the first open-identity option enabling interested adult donor-conceived persons to identify and possibly contact donors, potentially facilitating parental openness. Discussing donor conception openly—in contrast to historically common practices of secrecy—prevents the disruption associated with "late discovery" in adulthood and encourages children to feel comfortable about their origins, ultimately fostering positive psychological outcomes.[19] Consistent with the data, the American Society of Reproductive Medicine (ASRM) updated recommendations that providers encourage parents of donor-conceived persons disclose early and often,[20] and clarified its definition of "infertility" in 2023 to facilitate access to care for LGBTQ+ hopeful parents.[21]

NEXT, THE WARNING

The expansion of knowledge, human rights, and civil liberties underlying advances in public health and well-being are under threat.

We must take the authors and supporters of regressive policies at their word: the family is a unit of governance. Particularly following the *Dobbs* decision and the ensuing retrogression of reproductive rights, attacks on LGBTQ+ people must be understood—and resisted—as steps toward the goal of stripping the civil and human rights of women, minorities, and people with disabilities. Regressive and sexist policies restricting reproductive choice and targeting LGBTQ+ people—particularly gender minorities—have proliferated for years and have at their roots the harmful social structures of misogyny, heteronormativity, and cisnormativity.

These efforts to codify inequity have intensified to unprecedented levels in legislation, and related press and social media discourse advance patently unscientific claims that support eliminating abortion, abolishing gender, reducing sex to a binary by fiat, and codifying narrow definitions of terms such as "family," "mother," and "father," exacerbating vulnerabilities associated with outdated state parentage laws. To obscure the faulty bases and harmful impact of such policies, it is necessary to defund and devalue science and expertise in favor of misinformation and disinformation (i.e., "alternative facts"). Tellingly, the administration has moved to halt SOGIE data collection and research. The ultimate goal of these policies is to prevent LGBTQ+ people from full and open engagement in civic life. This crusade will not end with LGBTQ+ people. As the US Supreme Court recognized in *Bostock v Clayton County* (590 US 644 [2020]), sexism underlies homophobia and transphobia. This obsession with the immutable biological reality of sex serves to reinforce the reduction of women to reproductive and caregiving roles within nuclear families, threatening to roll back progress to a time—not so distant—when women were not recognized as full legal persons.

FINALLY, THE CALL TO ACTION

Professional organizations and individual professionals must speak and act to support the LGBTQ+ community and to defend science and science-based policy. In addition, public health professionals must support the modernization of state parentage laws to protect nongenetic family relationships.

Organizations Must Defend Science

It is crucial that reproductive and family policy incorporate gender-neutral language and expansive, inclusive definitions of terms such as "infertility" and "family." The leadership of organizations such as ASRM—which advocates on behalf of professionals and patients, funds multidisciplinary research, promotes ethical practice, and provides evidence-based information—is critical at this moment. For two decades, ASRM has consistently and repeatedly affirmed its support of providing assisted reproductive services to lesbian and gay hopeful parents. Ten years ago, ASRM similarly indicated support for transgender prospective parents, stating that "[p]rograms should treat all requests for assisted reproduction without regard to gender identity."[22(p1111)] When the White House issued an executive order in January 2025 declaring that the US government thenceforth would "recognize two sexes, male and female," and asserting that "gender identity . . . does not provide a meaningful basis for identification,"[23] ASRM responded swiftly, issuing a press release and evidence-based factsheet explaining gender and its differentiation from sex.[24] When the administration sought policy recommendations regarding IVF, ASRM expressed readiness to "engag[e] with the administration and Congress," and urged—based upon its "deep expertise"—that medical decisions should be "made by patients and physicians, not by bureaucrats, politicians, or insurance companies," that treatment should "meet . . . modern standards of care," and that policy solutions should be "inclusive of all patients who need care."[25]

While such professional policy statements are urgently necessary, simply letting people through the clinic door is not enough. Providing ethical, evidence-based care to sexual and gender minority patients requires population-specific data collection and research. For example, applying routine infertility treatment protocols to same-sex female couples seeking donor conception substantially increases risk during pregnancy without significantly increasing the likelihood of achieving pregnancy.[5] It is important for professional organizations to step forward to ensure that SOGIE data collection and cross-disciplinary research continue and to respond swiftly and decisively to disingenuous efforts to mischaracterize research documenting the negative impacts of discrimination and minority stress. Crucially, groups that historically have supported and worked in coalition with the LGBTQ+ community must not abandon us in this critical moment by cheerleading carve-outs for IVF in policies that erode reproductive rights or that expand access to reproductive health care for a subset of "desirable" prospective parents.

State Parentage Laws Must Protect Nongenetic Families

We and countless others have documented the flourishing of LGBTQ+ families, finding consistently that despite coping with prejudice and minority stress, children raised in these families are at least as healthy and resilient as children raised in so-called "traditional" families. Given the consistent and compelling body of evidence accumulated over decades demonstrating positive outcomes for children born through assisted reproduction reared by LGBTQ+ parents, it is deeply troubling that LGBTQ+ family advocacy organizations such as Children of Lesbians and Gays Everywhere (COLAGE) must continue to fight for parentage reform, even in the wake of US Supreme Court decisions legalizing same-sex marriage nationwide and guaranteeing same-sex married couples the full rights and privileges of marriage. Parentage, the legal relationship between parent and child, establishes crucial rights and responsibilities. Outdated laws in numerous US states fail to provide simple, accessible pathways for genetically unrelated parents to secure their legal relationships to their children, subjecting many to costly, intrusive processes such as adoptive "home studies."[4] This leaves many genetically unrelated parents and their children vulnerable in contexts such as divorce, the death of a genetically related parent, or family policing system involvement.

Few heterosexual parents are obliged to adopt their children born through assisted reproduction or to travel with copies of marriage and birth certificates to ensure their family relationships will be recognized in emergencies. Few children of heterosexual parents feel compelled to vigilantly consider whether, when, and with whom to share information about their families to avoid discrimination. These unfortunately common experiences for LGBTQ+ families underline the urgent need to enact legislation such as the Uniform Parentage Act (2017), which recognizes the diverse ways modern families are formed and creates clear, accessible pathways to parentage.[26] Children should not have to fear losing their parents and siblings, nor parents fear separation from children they planned for, care for, and desperately love—their "pride and joy."

Individual Actions as a Form of Support

Individuals researching and working with LGBTQ+ individuals and families and all those tasked with the promotion of public health must stand up and stand fast in the current moment. The following are actions they must take to accomplish this:

- First and foremost, treat LGBTQ+ individuals and families with dignity and respect: use gender-inclusive language.
- Model allyship by sharing pronouns.
- Avoid making assumptions about familial relationships or structure, including that genetic ties are necessary for relationships to be "real" or healthy.
- Build coalitions; bring an intersectional and interdisciplinary lens to gender, reproduction, and family.
- Refuse to anticipate or comply with discriminatory policies, particularly capricious diktats unlikely to survive legal challenges.
- Connect with local advocates.
- Show up to actions, advocacy, and community-building events.
- Harness expertise in op-eds and legislative testimony.
- Contact representatives to support modernizing outdated parentage laws.
- Challenge narratives that privilege some families while pathologizing others.
- Oppose discriminatory laws intended to restrict the rights of LGBTQ+ people and policies that hinder or selectively facilitate reproductive choice and access to health care.

- Support policies that promote self-determination and reproductive choice for all.

Everyone should be free to determine and pursue their own family building plans, including whether, when, how, and with whom to build a family. AJPH

CORRESPONDENCE

Correspondence should be sent to Sonja Mackenzie, Associate Professor and Chair, Department of Public Health, Santa Clara University, 500 El Camino Real, Santa Clara, CA 95053 (e-mail: smackenzie@scu.edu). Reprints can be ordered at https://ajph.org by clicking the "Reprints" link.

PUBLICATION INFORMATION

Full Citation: Mackenzie S, Johnson NN, Scheib JE, Kali L, Wilson J. Flourishing families: promoting public health and reproductive justice for all by protecting and supporting LGBTQ+ families in policy and practice. *Am J Public Health*. 2026;116(2): 197–201.

Acceptance Date: July 28, 2025.

DOI: https://doi.org/10.2105/AJPH.2025.308262

ORCID iDs:

Sonja Mackenzie https://orcid.org/0000-0002-9163-576X

Nesta N. Johnson https://orcid.org/0009-0007-7139-1669

Joanna E. Scheib https://orcid.org/0000-0003-4767-1146

Liam Kali https://orcid.org/0009-0003-3479-0725

CONTRIBUTORS

S. Mackenzie led this project. All authors contributed equally to the policy analysis and arguments of this piece. S. Mackenzie and N. N. Johnson were the primary researchers and authors of the first two drafts. J. E. Scheib, L. Kali, and J. Wilson conducted substantive research, writing, and editing. N. N. Johnson contributed primary editing throughout.

CONFLICTS OF INTEREST

The authors have no conflicts of interest to disclose.

REFERENCES

1. Xu W. The US administration assault on global reproductive health and autonomy. *Health Hum Rights*. 2025;27(1):95–99. Available at: https://www.hhrjournal.org/2025/02/13/the-us-administration-assault-on-global-reproductive-health-and-autonomy. Accessed March 18, 2025.
2. The White House. President Donald J. Trump expands access to in vitro fertilization (IVF). February 18, 2025. Available at: https://www.whitehouse.gov/fact-sheets/2025/02/fact-sheet-president-donald-j-trump-expands-access-to-in-vitro-fertilization-ivf. Accessed March 18, 2025.
3. Hendrickson J. Vivek Ramaswamy's truth. *The Atlantic.* August 21, 2023. Available at: https://www.theatlantic.com/politics/archive/2023/08/vivek-ramaswamy-gop-election/675041. Accessed March 12, 2025.
4. Movement Advancement Project. *Relationships at Risk: Why We Need to Update State Parentage Laws to Protect Children and Families*. 2023. Available at: https://www.mapresearch.org/2023-parentage-report. Accessed March 12, 2025.
5. Kali L. Therapeutic donor insemination for LGBTQ+ families: a systematic review. *Fertil Steril.* 2024;122(5):783–788. https://doi.org/10.1016/j.fertnstert.2024.08.347
6. Valido A, Harbour V, Scheib JE. Increase in open-identity sperm donation in the United States since 1996. *Fertil Steril.* 2025;123(2):361–363. https://doi.org/10.1016/j.fertnstert.2024.09.012
7. Mackenzie S. Bio-genetics and/at the border: the structural intimacies of LGBTQ transnational kinship. In: Boydell V, Dow K, eds. *Technologies of Reproductive Across the Lifecourse: Expanding Reproductive Studies.* Emerald Studies in Reproduction, Culture and Society. Bingley, UK: Emerald Publishing Limited; 2022. https://doi.org/10.1108/978-1-80071-733-620221014
8. Krug H. 2024 Board of Health Request for Rule-making for Gamete Bank and Fertility Clinic Programs 5 CCR 1005-6, Donor Conceived Persons and Gamete Agencies, Gamete Banks, and Fertility Clinics. Colorado Department of Public Health. 2024. Available at: https://www.sos.state.co.us/CCR/Upload/NoticeOfRulemaking/ProposedRuleAttach2024-00365.pdf. Accessed March 20, 2025.
9. Luterman S, Sosin K. A lesbian mom raised her son for two years. An Oklahoma judge erased that in 15 minutes. *The 19th.* May 20, 2022. Available at: https://19thnews.org/2022/05/oklahoma-custody-case-lgbtq-parenting-marriage-equality. Accessed March 21, 2025.
10. Kali KL. *Queer Conception: The Complete Fertility Guide for Queer and Trans Parents to Be*. Seattle, WA: Sasquatch Books; 2022.
11. Merriam-Webster. "Pride": the word that went from vice to strength. Available at: https://www.merriam-webster.com/wordplay/pride-meaning-word-history. Accessed March 18, 2025.
12. Vinney C. Experts reveal the one key difference between joy and happiness. October 30, 2024. *Verywell Mind.* Available at: https://www.verywellmind.com/joy-vs-happiness-8724682. Accessed March 18, 2025.
13. Bronski M. *A Queer History of the United States.* Boston, MA: Beacon Press; 2012.
14. Weston K. *Families We Choose: Lesbians, Gays, Kinship.* New York, NY: Columbia University Press; 1991.
15. Center for American Progress. Expanding definitions of family in federal laws. 2020. Available at: https://www.americanprogress.org/article/expanding-definitions-family-federal-laws. Accessed September 26, 2025.
16. Wilson BDM, Bouton LJA. LGBTQ parenting in the US. Williams Institute. July 2024. Available at: https://williamsinstitute.law.ucla.edu/publications/lgbt-parenting-us. Accessed March 9, 2025.
17. Hailey J, Burton W, Arscott J. We are family: chosen and created families as a protective factor against racialized trauma and anti-LGBTQ oppression among African American sexual and gender minority youth. *J GLBT Fam Stud.* 2020;16(2):176–191. https://doi.org/10.1080/1550428X.2020.1724133
18. Imrie S, Golombok S. Impact of new family forms on parenting and child development. *Annu Rev Dev Psychol*. 2020;2:295–316. https://doi.org/10.1146/annurev-devpsych-070220-122704
19. Carone N, Koh AS, Bos HMW, Rothblum ED, Gartrell NK. Two decades of psychological adjustment of donor-conceived offspring of lesbian parents: examining donor contact and type. *Reprod Biomed Online.* 2025;51(4):105020. https://doi.org/10.1016/j.rbmo.2025.105020
20. American Society for Reproductive Medicine. Reproductive facts: gamete and embryo donation: deciding whether to tell. 2021. Available at: https://www.reproductivefacts.org/globalassets/_rf/news-and-publications/bookletsfact-sheets/english-pdf/gamete_donation_deciding_whether_to_tell-factsheet.pdf. Accessed March 21, 2025.
21. American Society for Reproductive Medicine Practice Committee. Definition of infertility: a committee opinion. 2023. Available at: https://www.asrm.org/practice-guidance/practice-committee-documents/denition-of-infertility. Accessed March 20, 2025.
22. Ethics Committee of the American Society for Reproductive Medicine. Access to fertility services by transgender persons: an Ethics Committee opinion. *Fertil Steril.* 2015;104(5):1111–1115. https://doi.org/10.1016/j.fertnstert.2015.08.021
23. The White House. Defending Women From Gender Ideology Extremism and Restoring Biological Truth to the Federal Government. January 20, 2025. Available at: https://www.whitehouse.gov/presidential-actions/2025/01/defending-women-from-gender-ideology-extremism-and-restoring-biological-truth-to-the-federal-government. Accessed October 5, 2025.
24. American Society for Reproductive Medicine. Just the facts: biological sex. Available at: https://www.asrm.org/advocacy-and-policy/fact-sheets-and-one-pagers/just-the-facts-biological-sex. Accessed March 12, 2025.
25. American Society for Reproductive Medicine. Just the facts: IVF policy priorities. Available at: https://www.asrm.org/globalassets/_asrm/advocacy-and-policy/advocacy-resources/just-the-facts-ivf-policy-priorities.pdf. Accessed March 12, 2025.
26. Uniform Law Commission. Parentage Act. 2017. Available at: https://www.uniformlaws.org/committees/community-home?CommunityKey=c4f37d2d-4d20-4be0-8256-22dd73af068f. Accessed March 20, 2025.

Celebrating the Legacy and Urgency of Sex-Positive, Queer-Led Public Health

Scott D. Rhodes, PhD, MPH

ABOUT THE AUTHOR

The author is with the Department of Social Sciences and Health Policy, Wake Forest University School of Medicine, Winston-Salem, NC.

See also LGBTQ+ Well-Being and Joy, pp. 188–250.

The analytic essay by Adrian et al. (p. 214) honors the radical legacy of early community-led HIV prevention efforts, most notably those of Gay Men's Health Crisis (GMHC), and draws important connections to contemporary queer-affirming public health practice. As a gay man who has spent decades working at the intersections of lesbian, gay, bisexual, transgender, and queer (LGBTQ+) health; HIV prevention; and community-engaged research, I find this essay deeply affirming and instructive as well as a critical reminder of the profound legacy that informs our current efforts. The early days of the HIV epidemic that the authors describe sparked my own commitment to public health and led me to long-term collaborations with queer communities in the United States, Guatemala, and the Caribbean.

Adrian et al. remind us of what public health at its best can look like: bold, community driven, culturally responsive, and defiant in the face of stigma and government inaction. Their work recovers a history too often minimized or sterilized by dominant narratives, particularly those that downplay the roles of community, pleasure, and eroticism in the fight against HIV. The early epidemic was not only a public health emergency; it was also a moment of grassroots mobilization and organization that fundamentally reshaped the meaning of intimacy, solidarity, and resilience within queer communities.

Adrian and colleagues' essay is especially timely given the current climate of renewed anti-LGBTQ+ rhetoric, legislative assaults on bodily autonomy, and persistent health inequities. It serves as both a tribute and a call to action, challenging today's public health professionals, including researchers like me, to remember the radical roots of HIV prevention and to recommit ourselves to centering queer lives, histories, and strengths in our work.

QUEER RESISTANCE AS PUBLIC HEALTH

The essay's archival and oral history sources illustrate how GMHC and other early AIDS service organizations understood that survival depended on rejecting shame. These community groups built a model of health promotion and disease prevention that did not frame sex as a risk but rather as a source of connection, joy, and political power. Their campaigns did not rely on fear or judgment; they prioritized authenticity, community, and lived experience. The authors' framing of these campaigns within the themes of gay liberation, community connectedness, and eroticism is apt and instructive.

In my own research conducted in partnership with community members and organizations, we have likewise centered lived experience and social connection as tools to promote health and well-being. In our Appalachian Access Project, for example, trained community-based peer navigators, from the same queer communities they serve, harness in-person and mHealth social media to deliver targeted, tailored, and personalized messages that affirm identities and offer practical support for accessing and using prevention and care services. These services include those related to HIV, sexually transmitted infection, hepatitis C virus, and mpox testing; preexposure prophylaxis (PrEP), syringe service programs, and mpox vaccinations; care and treatment for HIV, sexually transmitted infections, hepatitis C virus, and mpox; and medically supervised gender-affirming care.[1] The intervention draws directly from community insight and leverages community strengths, just as GMHC's earliest efforts did.

As noted by Adrian et al., sex-positive approaches are not without controversy. GMHC's use of explicit language and erotic imagery drew fire from both within and outside queer communities. Senator Jesse Helms's infamous 1987 tirade against GMHC's "Safer Sex Comix" is a stark reminder that pleasure-centered public health has long been political. And yet, despite federal funding cuts and moral panic, these campaigns persisted because they were unapologetically of the community. They were also highly successful in reaching at-risk communities with accessible, culturally responsive messaging as well as changing risk behaviors such as condomless anal sex.[2,3]

CONTEMPORARY ECHOES AND ENDURING LESSONS

Adrian et al. also link early sex-positive prevention efforts to present-day efforts such as PrEP4Love,[4] We Prevent,[5] and 2GETHER,[6] interventions that likewise affirm pleasure, intimacy, and community as central to sexual health. In community-engaged research that I conducted in partnership with Latine immigrant communities and with queer people in rural Appalachia,[7–9] I have witnessed the transformative power of interventions and programs that meet people where they are and speak to their realities—who they are and what they value—not simply their sexual risks. The Appalachian Access Project is not just about connecting people to PrEP, for example; it is about creating a space where queer persons in rural Appalachia can see themselves, their values, and their desires reflected. Peer navigators meet people where they live, in kitchens, on porches, at drag nights, and through direct messaging, transforming prevention and care from a lecture about risk into informal intimate conversations about communities, belonging, resilience, and pleasure.

Whether we are promoting PrEP or doxycycline postexposure prophylaxis use, undetectable equals untransmittable, harm reduction strategies, or regular screening for HIV and other sexually transmitted infections, the principles outlined in the Adrian et al. essay remain core to success, including affirming identity, building community, and celebrating pleasure. Our work with interventions such as ChiCAS (a culturally responsive small-group intervention for transgender Latinas)[8] and HOLA en Grupos (a community-based peer navigation intervention for Spanish-speaking gay, bisexual, and other men who have sex with men and for Spanish-speaking transgender women)[9] reinforces what GMHC demonstrated decades ago: effective health promotion must be grounded in the culture, values, and language of the communities it aims to affect. It must be engaging, affirming, and, yes, even fun and sexy.

Adrian et al. also push us to understand queer public health as something more expansive than disease prevention. It is about creating space for LGBTQ+ people to feel valued, understood, and connected. Today, queer communities continue to experience the compounded effects of homonegativity, transnegativity, racism, xenophobia, and stigma based on intersecting identities. Sex-positive, culturally responsive, and community-driven public health programs are not optional; they are essential.

A RESEARCH AGENDA ROOTED IN PRIDE

Adrian and colleagues' essay also calls for renewed scholarly attention to the roles of liberation, collective responsibility, and eroticism in contemporary HIV prevention. Too often, public health research still marginalizes or sanitizes queer experience in the name of "neutrality" or "generalizability." But as Adrian et al. demonstrate (and my work affirms), queer joy, pleasure, and kinship are not only worthy of study but can be essential to health promotion and disease prevention.

Moving forward, we need more research that centers queer epistemologies and lived experience. We also need to expand our understanding of how cultural context and grassroots expertise inform successful interventions and programs. Importantly, we must ensure that these investigations are inclusive of transgender and nonbinary people, queer people of color, people who use substances, and others who have long been underserved or excluded by traditional public health.

CONCLUSION

Adrian et al. have given us more than a historical case study; they have given us a framework to renew our thinking critically and expansively about public health practice and research today. They invite us to see HIV prevention not just as a technical endeavor but as an act of love, resistance, power, voice, and affirmation. In doing so, they challenge all of us to center community wisdom, uplift marginalized voices, and lead with pride, bravery, and joy. For those of us working in queer health, HIV prevention, public health, and research, this essay is more than a reflection on the past. It is a reminder of the path we walk, a path forged by courage, creativity, and an unwavering belief that our lives, our love, and our pleasure matter. AJPH

CORRESPONDENCE

Correspondence should be sent to Scott D. Rhodes, PhD, MPH, Medical Center Boulevard, Department of Social Sciences and Health Policy, Wake Forest University School of Medicine, Winston-Salem, NC 27157 (e-mail: srhodes@wakehealth.edu). Reprints can be ordered at https://www.ajph.org by clicking the "Reprints" link.

AJPH February 2026, Vol. 116, No. 2

PUBLICATION INFORMATION

Full Citation: Rhodes SD. Celebrating the legacy and urgency of sex-positive, queer-led public health. *Am J Public Health*. 2026;116(2):202–204.

Acceptance Date: August 26, 2025.

DOI: https://doi.org/10.2105/AJPH.2025.308286

ORCID iD:
Scott D. Rhodes https://orcid.org/0000-0002-9797-8114

ACKNOWLEDGMENTS

I gratefully acknowledge the extraordinary queer-serving community organizations and partners who have placed their trust in me and with whom I have had the privilege of working for more than three decades.

Note. The findings and conclusions in this report are those of the author and do not necessarily represent the official position of the Wake Forest University School of Medicine.

CONFLICTS OF INTEREST

The author has no conflicts of interest.

REFERENCES

1. Rhodes SD, Tanner AE, Alonzo J, et al. Using ENGAGED for CHANGE to develop a multicultural intervention to reduce disparities among sexual and gender minorities in Appalachia. *Prog Community Health Partnersh*. 2024;18(4):447–458. Available at: https://pmc.ncbi.nlm.nih.gov/articles/PMC12186249. Accessed September 19, 2025.
2. Greenblatt J. The banality of anal: safer sexual erotics in the Gay Men's Health Crisis' Safer Sex Comix and Ex Aequo's Alex et la vie d'après. *J Med Humanit*. 2019;40(1):33–51. https://doi.org/10.1007/s10912-018-9535-z
3. Rakower J, Hallyburton A. Disease information through comics: a graphic option for health education. *J Med Humanit*. 2022;43(3):475–492. https://doi.org/10.1007/s10912-022-09730-9
4. Phillips G, Raman AB, Felt D, et al. PrEP4Love: the role of messaging and prevention advocacy in PrEP attitudes, perceptions, and uptake among YMSM and transgender women. *J Acquir Immune Defic Syndr*. 2020;83(5):450–456. https://doi.org/10.1097/qai.0000000000002297
5. Gamarel KE, Darbes LA, Wall KM, et al. A relationship-focused HIV prevention intervention for young sexual minority men in the United States: a pilot randomized controlled trial of the We Prevent Intervention. *AIDS Behav*. 2023;27(8):2703–2719. https://doi.org/10.1007/s10461-023-03994-5
6. Newcomb ME, Swann G, Addington EL, et al. Randomized controlled trial of a relationship education and HIV prevention program for young male couples: biomedical and behavioral outcomes. *Health Psychol*. 2025;44(3):297–309. https://doi.org/10.1037/hea0001448
7. Rhodes SD, Mann L, Siman FM, et al. ENGAGED for CHANGE: an innovative community-based participatory research strategy to intervention development. In: Wallerstein N, Duran B, Oetzel J, Minkler M, eds. *Community-Based Participatory Research for Health*. 3rd ed. Jossey-Bass; 2017: 189–202.
8. Rhodes SD, Alonzo J, Mann-Jackson L, et al. Preexposure prophylaxis uptake among Spanish-speaking transgender women: a randomized controlled trial in North and South Carolina, 2019–2022. *Am J Public Health*. 2024;114(1):68–78. https://doi.org/10.2105/ajph.2023.307444
9. Rhodes SD, Alonzo J, Mann L, et al. Small-group randomized controlled trial to increase condom use and HIV testing among Hispanic/Latino gay, bisexual, and other men who have sex with men. *Am J Public Health*. 2017;107(6):969–976.

"It Has Transformed Living for Me": The Trajectory of Alignment, Comfort, and Social Connectedness After Gender-Affirming Surgery

Tyler Gaedecke, RN, PhD, Kasey Jackman, RN, PhD, Maureen George, RN, PhD, Miriam Ryvicker, PhD, and Walter Bockting, PhD

See also LGBTQ+ Well-Being and Joy, pp. 188–250.

Gender-affirming surgery can reduce distress about gender incongruence among transgender and gender-diverse adults, contributing to improved mental health and quality of life. However, a greater understanding of the psychosocial changes after surgery that influence well-being is needed to maximize these outcomes. In this analysis of interviews (conducted in New York City, January 2023–February 2025) with individuals in the first year after gender-affirming surgery, we identified one such mechanism: an increased sense of connection to one's body fosters the stability, comfort, and environmental awareness to live freely and connect with others. (*Am J Public Health.* 2026;116(2): 205–209. https://doi.org/10.2105/AJPH.2025.308263)

AJPH February 2026, Vol. 116, No. 2

For much of the transgender and gender-diverse (TGD) population (i.e., those whose gender identity differs from the sex they were assigned at birth), gender-affirming mental and physical health care is an important part of health promotion across the life span.[1] Although individuals' care needs vary, some may seek surgery that alters primary or secondary sex characteristics to align their body with their gender identity. The beneficial impact of gender-affirming surgeries on mental health and quality of life for the TGD adults who obtain them has been established.[2,3]

Beyond those positive findings, data about patients' expected and experienced outcomes of gender-affirming surgery are still lacking depth and individualization.[4,5] For example, questions remain about which outcomes of surgery are experienced by TGD people as most influential to their overall quality of life. Research centering gender minority stress[6,7] and gender dysphoria[1] (i.e., distress attributable to gender incongruence) helps researchers, clinicians, and TGD communities describe and explain the unique psychological stressors faced by TGD people. However, there is a need for greater evidence about the mechanisms by which gender-affirming interventions foster life satisfaction and a sustainable sense of identity fulfillment.[8]

STUDY OBJECTIVE

The objective of our larger study was to better understand psychosocial well-being and quality of life in a prospective cohort of TGD adults after gender-affirming surgery. Because body image is one domain of well-being that may be expected to improve after surgery,[9] we asked qualitative interview participants how surgery changed their feelings about their body (if at all). Informed by participants' positive responses to this question, we sought to characterize what made their surgery feel beneficial to them. We present findings that contribute most directly to our understanding of the mechanisms through which gender-affirming surgery fosters improved quality of life.

RESEARCH QUESTION

How is improved body image experienced by TGD adults in the first year after gender-affirming surgery?

PARTICIPANTS, SAMPLE, GEOGRAPHIC LOCATION, SETTING, AND YEAR OF STUDY

We purposively selected this sample (n = 49) for the qualitative aim of our longitudinal, mixed methods cohort study (n = 300). We collected data from January 2023 to February 2025. Participants' mean age was 35.0 years (SD = 10.1; 18–64 years). The sample was 14% Black/African American (n = 7), 65% White (n = 32), 16% Asian (n = 8), and 27% Hispanic/Latino adults (n = 13); one non-Hispanic participant reported an "other" race. Of the sample, 20% was transmasculine (n = 10), 71% was transfeminine (n = 35), and 8% was nonbinary (n = 4).

We recruited participants following admission to a home visiting nurse program in New York City designed to provide care immediately after gender-affirming surgery. The most common surgery was vaginoplasty (n = 39; 80%), followed by metoidioplasty (n = 6; 12%) and phalloplasty (n = 4; 8%). We excluded facial feminization surgery patients from this analysis given facial surgery's unique social visibility. We did not include chest surgery patients in the sample because their recovery infrequently led to home care referral.

METHODS

Participants completed semistructured individual interviews via Zoom (Zoom Communications, San Jose, CA) 3 to 12 months after surgery. The interview guide, coding, and interpretations were informed by qualitative descriptive methodologies.[10] Audio-recorded interviews were transcribed professionally, and an interdisciplinary team of four individuals analyzed cleaned transcripts by using a conventional content analysis approach.[11] We iteratively developed a codebook through inductive, independent coding of the first 15 interviews before finalizing it and applying it to the remaining interviews. We addressed conflicts in weekly meetings, which an expert in qualitative research adjudicated. We present findings from a noteworthy coding category that captured how participants described their current relationship with their body and how it related to experiences of incongruence and related distress.

KEY FINDINGS

The analysis reflected two cross-cutting themes. The first theme, "I Feel Like I Landed," describes the sense of alignment that participants experienced after surgery, creating a sense of ease and relief that they had not previously known. Example quotations are presented in Box 1. Participants actively felt more present in their bodies but also described the passive luxury of no longer having to "think twice" about their bodies in their daily lives and said that they could finally "take a deep breath."

BOX 1— Exemplars for Theme 1: "I Feel Like I Landed"

"I mean, it's made my body look the way it felt already, right? . . . It's not something that I get reminded of; it feels natural, and it feels like how things are supposed to be. And that's really nice." (Participant 3, transgender woman)
"Just looking at my body in the mirror, liking what I see. For me in this moment, that's really it. My body matches my mind . . . . My body looks like who I know I am." (Participant 16, transmasculine)
"It's brought relief from my dysphoria in a way that I can't quantify because it's so big. . . . When I woke up from surgery, it was like somebody had taken the moon off of my back." (Participant 27, woman)
"Before [surgery], since I was misaligned, even if I need to take a shower or something, it's going to remind you of that. That you're different from others. You're just not you. After [surgery], I can see myself as a whole. So, it helps a lot." (Participant 6, feminine)
"My feelings about my physical body, oh my gosh. I feel like a goddess. I feel like I landed. I feel like I finally have a shell that reflects the ghost inside of me." (Participant 13, female)
"[Dysphoria] is something I don't constantly obsess about and worry about. . . . That's been the biggest change; it's just a higher level of comfort with my body. . . . [I feel] far more steady. I'm less explosive . . . more confident." (Participant 5, female)
"I felt like I was in a dream; I was dreamin' the whole time and this is the real body I was in all the time." (Participant 25, female)
"My brain very clearly, as it has all of my life, had a very clear image of who I am and the mirror never quite lined up with that image. But, so doing surgery just really helped the schema align a little bit better." (Participant 45, male)
"You feel, of course, more confident, but it makes me more happy about life in general. . . . I feel like I was born again; when [I had] that surgery, I feel like my life changed completely and I feel very happy." (Participant 38, transgender woman)
"I was very dysphoric. . . . I had that feeling since I was a teenager, from like 12 to 25, 26. . . . [Now, I'm] mentally way, way better. As I described it to my therapist, my dysphoria has gone down at least by 90%." (Participant 44, transgender male)

Note. Gender identities mentioned reflect participants' self-described gender.

The second theme, "I'm Experiencing the World," describes newfound life possibilities and awareness (of themselves and their environments) after surgery. Example quotations are presented in Box 2. The alignment following surgery provided them with confidence and a new sense of access to experiences they did not previously feel comfortable with, giving them the chance to "try the life [they had] always wanted."

Importantly, these two themes were interconnected. Participants reinforced the notion that being connected with one's body (theme 1) was the foundation on which they experienced new and exciting experiences, social connection, and self-improvement (theme 2):

> I didn't realize how life-changing it would be to have this surgery . . . and how much more comfortable it would make me. That, in turn, has made it easier for me to focus on bettering my health in different ways. . . . Even though I'm not entirely where I wanna be yet, this felt like such a huge step forward. . . . I do at this moment feel a lot more connected to my body. (Participant 21, transgender man)

> It wasn't a matter of stigma, but rather a matter of the lack of dysphoria that made me feel more at ease in my environment, and I think that showed. . . . So honestly, I found that after surgery, interacting with people became a lot easier. And I think a big part of it is I find myself more present in the moment and not stuck up in my head the entire time. (Participant 27, woman)

> My whole body, I mean, it's realigned. Before, I wasn't really in my body. . . . I had a real cerebral experience up until a certain point. Since the surgery, I'm in my body. I'm having not just an experience of my mind but also of my body now, and that's great. I feel it, I feel at home, I'm experiencing the world, our society, our culture, my neighborhood, and myself far better, more accurately now. I'm experiencing it with less challenges, less barriers. I couldn't before, and now I can. . . . It's transformed living for me. (Participant 23, female)

EVALUATION, TRANSFERABILITY, AND ADVERSE EFFECTS

Our participants' responses identified concepts that exceed the notion of body image alone. Many responses were not explicitly about gender and reflected a broader confidence associated with a more fully integrated sense of self. The impacts of surgery quickly manifested in a deeply felt relief that made room for fun, connection, and a sense of control. These experiences also crystallized their presurgery experience: they were not "in" their body before, but now they are, and they are enjoying it. This shift in locus of control helped some participants engage in new habits for self-care and health promotion, further emphasizing the potential value of gender-affirming surgery for everyday life and long-term well-being.

BOX 2— Exemplars for Theme 2: "I'm Experiencing the World"

"Before [surgery], I felt shameful, like I had this secret or something. I was afraid to do certain things. . . . I never felt comfortable doing that, like going to Pilates classes, going to the beach, or going to the spa with my friends and stuff like that. But now I feel comfortable to be able to do all those things." (Participant 28, transgender woman)
"I just sort of pushed away thinking about my body . . . but now I'm like, oh, no, I'm pretty. I love me. I want to take care of me, and so, I do a lot more yoga. . . . I'm enjoying setting health goals for myself because they're also helping me pick up new hobbies that previously would have hit my dysphoria. . . . It's very much allowing me to take care of my body in a way that I didn't care to before." (Participant 20, transgender woman)
"I feel like it's also just made me less self-conscious about even things that are unrelated. . . . I stopped shaving [my legs] and my armpits, which I feel like I would have had more of an issue with before. . . . I'm much more fine with that." (Participant 2, nonbinary)
"My girlfriend doesn't care one way or the other, but like, being able to be intimate without [dysphoria] being something that's always in the back of my mind." (Participant 3, transgender woman)
"I've worked so hard to get to the baseline where everybody else is with their body, and then I'll do other normal people things, like work, think about my job and my relationships, and all that. But, yeah, I'm very close to that [after surgery]. And I'm trying to, I don't know, worry about things that aren't related to being transgender anymore." (Participant 47, transgender man)
"When you have something on you that you know isn't supposed to be there and your brain is telling you it's not supposed to be there, it's constantly getting in the way of things you want to do. . . . I finally feel like I can go through my day without having to worry, 'How does this look on me,' 'How do I feel in these clothes.'. . . It's so much easier, and those aspects of life I am able to enjoy so much more." (Participant 15, transgender woman)
"There was, like, the world's largest bounce house that came nearby a couple of months ago . . . and I had the most fun ever. It was the best experience ever. And then, I realized halfway through, I could not be enjoying this right now if I hadn't had this surgery. I am so glad I had this surgery . . . and I was able to do this thing." (Participant 12, gender fluid)

Note. Gender identities mentioned here reflect participants' self-described gender.

Limitations of our study include the potential that social desirability bias led participants to respond in a manner meant to please the researchers. Furthermore, this sample comprised primarily vaginoplasty patients, so our findings are not necessarily transferable to individuals receiving other gender-affirming surgeries. The study was also necessarily limited to the perspectives of TGD individuals who sought and could access surgery. The 3- to 12-month postoperative time frame may have also introduced time-varying responses between participants, and some outcomes may not yet be clear after 12 months. Nevertheless, our findings describe the relief of distress and a shift in embodiment affecting both one's sense of self and one's place in the world.

Participants also described challenges and adjustments in this postoperative period as they learned about their changed anatomy, including surgical complications or discrepancies between expectations and results.[4,12] However, stressors associated with any significant life change may exist in the postoperative period regardless of outcome.[5] The conceptualization of "success" in gender-affirming surgery often emphasizes the impact on mental health; however, our findings indicate that mental health and quality of life may be indirectly improved through the mediating direct outcomes of reduced dysphoria or incongruence and improved connection to body, self, and others, facilitating both identity and intimacy. Therefore, in addition to mental health, alignment with one's body, sense of self, and interpersonal efficacy may be important outcomes to assess.[9,13]

SCALABILITY

Scalability is not applicable to this study.

PUBLIC HEALTH SIGNIFICANCE

These findings illuminate the diverse yet overwhelmingly positive experiences that were made possible for these participants who obtained the gender-affirming surgery they were seeking. Participants' vivid descriptions may also help researchers and clinicians reimagine and expand on the measurement of mental health outcomes after gender-affirming care, as surgery might be one of several milestones in a lifelong process of TGD identity development rather than the finish line.[4,14] Future research on embodiment (i.e., understanding how TGD individuals achieve internal and external congruence)[15] could develop these ideas further and improve support before and after surgery. For now, a clear case is present for clinicians to ensure that gender-affirming surgery is available and accessible to the adults who seek it. AJPH

ABOUT THE AUTHORS

Tyler Gaedecke, Kasey Jackman, Maureen George, and Walter Bockting are with the Center for Sexual and Gender Minority Health Research, Columbia University School of Nursing, New York, NY. Kasey Jackman is also with New York–Presbyterian Hospital, New York. Miriam Ryvicker is with the Center for Home Care Policy & Research, VNS Health, New York, NY. Walter Bockting is also with the New York State Psychiatric Institute/Columbia Psychiatry, New York.

CORRESPONDENCE

Correspondence should be sent to Tyler Gaedecke, Columbia University School of Nursing, 560 West 168th St, New York, NY 10032 (e-mail: tdg2123@cumc.columbia.edu). Reprints can be ordered at https://www.ajph.org by clicking the "Reprints" link.

PUBLICATION INFORMATION

Full Citation: Gaedecke T, Jackman K, George M, Ryvicker M, Bockting W. "It has transformed living for me": the trajectory of alignment, comfort, and social connectedness after gender-affirming surgery. *Am J Public Health*. 2026;116(2):205–209.

Acceptance Date: August 1, 2025.

DOI: https://doi.org/10.2105/AJPH.2025.308263

ORCID iD:
Tyler Gaedecke https://orcid.org/0009-0009-0694-6239

CONTRIBUTORS

T. Gaedecke conceptualized the article, led and participated in analyses, and led the writing. K. Jackman and M. George guided the study's implementation as coinvestigators. K. Jackman, M. George, M. Ryvicker, and W. Bockting provided critical feedback on early conceptualizations of the findings and reviewed and edited the article for clarity and coherence. M. George participated in and adjudicated qualitative analysis. M. Ryvicker and W. Bockting designed and supervised the research. All authors reviewed and approved the final version of the article.

ACKNOWLEDGMENTS

This research was supported by the National Institute of Nursing Research (NINR; grant R01NR019315; principal investigators: M. Ryvicker and W. Bockting; grant F31NR021239, principal investigator: T. Gaedecke).

The authors would like to acknowledge Skylar Hawthorne, LCSW, and Carolina Lopez for their contributions to the collection and coding of participant interviews and the members of the spring 2025 Gender and Sexuality Workshop at Columbia University Department of Sociology for feedback on early drafts and conceptualizations of this article.

Note. The contents of the article are solely the responsibility of the authors and do not necessarily represent the official views of NINR or the National Institutes of Health.

CONFLICTS OF INTEREST

The authors have no conflicts of interest to disclose.

HUMAN PARTICIPANT PROTECTION

This study was approved by two institutional review boards (IRBs): the VNS Health IRB (awarded institution and recruitment site; protocol I21-002) and the Columbia University IRB (Subawardee, site running qualitative arm; protocol AAAU0021).

REFERENCES

1. Coleman E, Radix AE, Bouman WP, et al. Standards of care for the health of transgender and gender diverse people, version 8. *Int J Transgend Health*. 2022;23(suppl 1):S1–S259. https://doi.org/10.1080/26895269.2022.2100644
2. Almazan AN, Keuroghlian AS. Association between gender-affirming surgeries and mental

health outcomes. *JAMA Surg.* 2021;156(7): 611–618. https://doi.org/10.1001/jamasurg.2021.0952

3. Murad MH, Elamin MB, Garcia MZ, et al. Hormonal therapy and sex reassignment: a systematic review and meta-analysis of quality of life and psychosocial outcomes. *Clin Endocrinol (Oxf).* 2010;72(2):214–231. https://doi.org/10.1111/j.1365-2265.2009.03625.x
4. Ross MB, Wesseling S, Mullender M, Kreukels BPC, van de Grift T. Expectations and experienced outcomes regarding gender-affirming surgeries: a pilot study. *Transgend Health.* 2024;9(4): 326–338. https://doi.org/10.1089/trgh.2022.0118
5. Oorthuys AOJ, Ross M, Kreukels BPC, Mullender MG, van de Grift T. Identifying coping strategies used by transgender individuals in response to stressors during and after gender-affirming treatments—an explorative study. *Healthcare (Basel).* 2022;11(1):89. https://doi.org/10.3390/healthcare11010089
6. Hendricks ML, Testa RJ. A conceptual framework for clinical work with transgender and gender nonconforming clients: an adaptation of the minority stress model. *Prof Psychol Res Pr.* 2012; 43(5):460–467. https://doi.org/10.1037/a0029597
7. Bockting W, Coleman E, Deutsch MB, et al. Adult development and quality of life of transgender and gender nonconforming people. *Curr Opin Endocrinol Diabetes Obes.* 2016;23(2):188–197. https://doi.org/10.1097/med.0000000000000232
8. Leitch J, Nguyen V, Potter S. Beyond dysphoria and stress: a theory of gender euphoria and gender fulfillment. *Int J Transgend Health.* 2025;9(1): 1–14. https://doi.org/10.1080/26895269.2024.2447786
9. Markey CH, Goodwin C, August KJ, et al. Exploring body image among transgender and nonbinary adults: considering positive body image and the pursuit of gender-affirming surgery. *J Health Psychol.* 2025;30(1):13591053241312509. https://doi.org/10.1177/13591053241312509
10. Bradshaw C, Atkinson S, Doody O. Employing a qualitative description approach in health care research. *Glob Qual Nurs Res.* 2017;4: 2333393617742282. https://doi.org/10.1177/2333393617742282
11. Hsieh HF, Shannon SE. Three approaches to qualitative content analysis. *Qual Health Res.* 2005;15(9):1277–1288. https://doi.org/10.1177/1049732305276687
12. Goetz TG, Arcomano AC. "Coming home to my body": a qualitative exploration of gender-affirming care-seeking and mental health. *J Gay Lesbian Ment Health.* 2023;27(4):380–400. https://doi.org/10.1080/19359705.2023.2237841
13. Bouman WP, Claes L, Brewin N, et al. Transgender and anxiety: a comparative study between transgender people and the general population. *Int J Transgend.* 2017;18(1):16–26. https://doi.org/10.1080/15532739.2016.1258352
14. Bockting W, Coleman E. Developmental stages of the transgender coming-out process: toward an integrated identity. In: Ettner R, Monstrey S, Coleman E, eds. *Principles of Transgender Medicine and Surgery.* 2nd ed. New York, NY: Routledge/Taylor & Francis Group; 2016:137–158.
15. Prosser J. *Second Skins: The Body Narratives of Transsexuality.* New York, NY: Columbia University Press; 1998.

Transgender Youth Health and Joy: A Model of Evidence-Based School District Policy Change to Support Transgender and Nonbinary Youth Health

Sonja Mackenzie, DrPH, ScM, Neha Mann, BS, and October Hertenstein

See also LGBTQ+ Well-Being and Joy, pp. 188–250.

There are 1000 antitransgender bills across the United States, more than one quarter of which target educational settings. School districts are an increasingly critical policy domain through which transgender and nonbinary youth health is harmed and can be protected. Trans-led resistance, including activism and advocacy, has been found to lead to improved health. This case study describes one California school district's policy advocacy process as a model for building transgender youth health through a participatory process that, in itself, has supported transgender joy. (*Am J Public Health*. 2026;116(2):210–213. https://doi.org/10.2105/AJPH.2025.308264)

AJPH February 2026, Vol. 116, No. 2

There are currently 1000 antitransgender bills under consideration across the United States, more than one quarter of which (27.3%) target educational settings through forcibly outing transgender students to parents, denying student autonomy in pronoun and name selection, banning gender education, and more.[1] Despite these policies' negative impacts on transgender youth health,[2–6] trans-led resistance, including activism and advocacy, has been documented to lead to improved health.[7–10] Since 2023, there have been six antitransgender bills introduced in California's State Assembly,[1] and more than a dozen school districts in California have introduced policies emulating antitransgender national and state bills.[11] In response, transgender youths have organized policy advocacy efforts in school districts throughout the state,[7,8,12] which are increasingly a key policy space for promoting transgender youth health.[13]

This article documents the process and outcomes of one district's work to create institutional and district-level policies to protect and promote transgender youth health. This collaborative effort responded to ongoing unmet needs identified by transgender and nonbinary youths in the district as antitransgender legislation increased throughout California. Students in this district's only public high school reported being unable to access bathrooms in a reliable manner, presenting health concerns. Transgender and nonbinary youths who experience bathroom discrimination demonstrate increased reporting of depressed mood and suicidal ideation.[5] Transgender and nonbinary students throughout the district reported ongoing bullying, reflective of national data that one in four transgender and nonbinary youths report being physically threatened or harmed in the past year.[4]

INTERVENTION AND IMPLEMENTATION

This project reflects the work of a Gender Equity Subcommittee (GES), one of two subcommittees formed as part of an ongoing effort initiated in 2022 when the school district's superintendent convened a Gender Equity and Sexual Harassment Advisory Committee to address transgender equity needs and prevent sexual harm. The GES project integrated collaboration between community and school stakeholders to support transgender health, well-being, and joy.

Monthly committee meetings facilitated by the school administrator and superintendent and monthly GES meetings took place online. These meetings supported issue identification, knowledge and resource sharing, and identification of potential solutions to address gender equity and transgender student health and well-being.

The following model for change identifies public health research, community advocacy, and transgender youth leadership (including power sharing) as interacting components for improving transgender equity, leading to environmental and policy changes in the district (Figure 1).

The GES started by establishing the evidence for the health and educational impacts of inadequate bathroom access and antitransgender bullying through conducting a literature review of peer-reviewed research using keywords of "transgender, youth, health, mental health, school, bathroom, bullying" on PubMed and PsycInfo published through 2024. Collaborations with local health professionals specializing in gender-affirming care and analysis of comparative school cases documented in reports and media publications allowed the GES to build on this research to compile a strong public health case.

Community advocacy took place through the presence of GES members and transgender student leaders who gave testimony at school board meetings. The involvement of key stakeholders across school levels (elementary, middle school, and high school) ensured that communications drew on and also fed back into school policy and practice. A central piece of this advocacy was the engagement of a school board member on the GES, who facilitated connection to policy resources and solutions. Through the establishment of a space for truly community-centered collaboration and power sharing centering transgender youths, administrators gained an enhanced understanding of transspecific concerns, and community members became aware of institutional and community resources for addressing barriers.

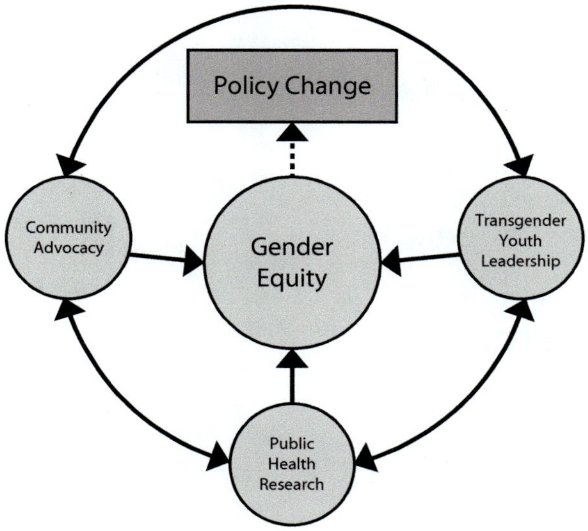

FIGURE 1— Gender Equity Model for Participatory Transgender Youth-Led Policy Change

Note. Public health research, community advocacy, and transgender youth leadership (including power sharing) are interacting components for improving transgender equity (solid lines), leading to environmental and policy changes in the district (dotted line).

Transgender and nonbinary youth leadership was the central and driving force of this project. High school students organized informal means of collecting narrative and visual documentation, including journals of bathroom access (or lack thereof) and impacts on health, and photos and videos of bathroom and school conditions. They also created schoolwide awareness campaigns (Figure 2).[14]

Students integrated evidence from public health research and gender-affirming mental health care to document the health impacts of lack of bathroom access. Students served as key facilitators of a process improvement assessment to identify transgender and nonbinary student needs. Students' persistence in bringing carefully organized visual and narrative documentation before the school board was key in centering the lived experience of impacted communities. In the words of one student advocate, testifying at a school board meeting in spring 2024, weeks after the death of nonbinary student Nex Benedict:

> Nex died because of an administration that did too little, too late. I see myself in Nex, another 16-year-old nonbinary person, another cook, another kid who liked rock music, another young American who had dreams. I need the problems with the bathrooms to be fixed before I lose my life or I lose one of my friends to this issue. I've had health problems associated with holding it all day, I've had other students tell me they feel unsafe walking into restrooms. –16-year-old nonbinary student

This year long effort led to three concrete outcomes: (1) one additional all-gender multistall restroom installed at

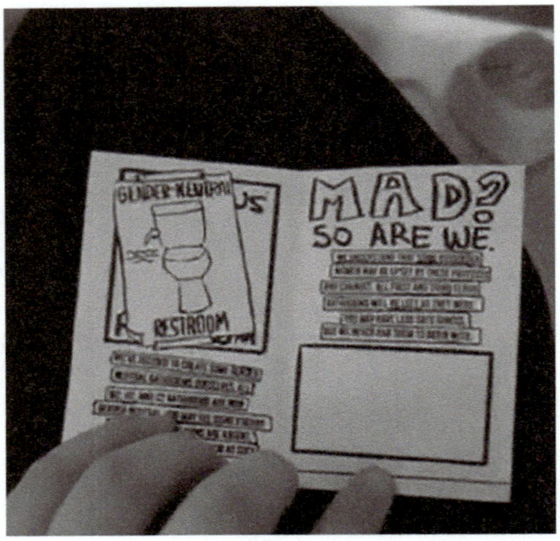

FIGURE 2— **Pages of Transgender Student Zine**

the high school, (2) a recommendations report that outlined evidence and need for further work, and (3) a district policy resolution in support of transgender and nonbinary students. This policy resolution was introduced by the school board member who had participated on the GES and was approved unanimously by the school board.

PLACE, TIME, AND PERSONS

The project period was from September 2023 to fall 2024 in an urban school district of more than 9000 K–12 students in California. The population targeted was the transgender and nonbinary students in the district and in particular at the high school for the bathroom inclusion objective. In 2022, surveys demonstrated an approximate estimate of 540 transgender and 450 nonbinary youths in the district (at 6% and 5%, respectively) in the middle and high schools.[14] Participants included the superintendent and Title IX coordinator, a parent representative from each school, a school board member, high school and middle school teachers, and transgender and nonbinary student leaders at the high school. The GES consisted of eight parents (including parents of transgender and nonbinary children), four teachers, two transgender and nonbinary students, and one undergraduate student research assistant.

PURPOSE

The goal of this community–school district collaboration was to identify opportunities for environmental change to support transgender and nonbinary student health and well-being. The objective was to draw on evidence and policy analysis to expand the availability and accessibility of all-gender restrooms at the high school.

EVALUATION AND ADVERSE EFFECTS

In evaluating the role of the GES in changing the policy and school-level environments for transgender youths, key stakeholders noted that the process (1) integrated public health evidence and principles into community advocacy strategies; (2) supported a genuine collaboration among community members, policy members, and school district leadership; and (3) centralized the leadership and needs of those with lived experience in the process of initiating institutional changes, in particular through the ongoing participation of transgender youths. We observed no adverse effects.

SUSTAINABILITY

Student organizers and community advocates alike must mentor ongoing leadership roles to ensure sustainability of these efforts and ongoing policy change. Threats to sustainability include the broader antitransgender political and public health context and threats to funding.

PUBLIC HEALTH SIGNIFICANCE

Nearly one in five people who identify as transgender are aged 13 to 17 years.[15] Trans-led organizing for policy change is an often-overlooked but necessary component of health promotion. Students at this high school are now able to access a safe all-gender bathroom and have the knowledge that, despite the broader political environment, the school district supports their right to exist and to be healthy.

Student organizers identified the critical importance of long-term trusted relationships with school leaders and teachers on their identity development and health. This underscores the necessity and lasting health impacts of transinclusive teacher training and inclusive practices among school administration. In light of the policy resolution affirming transgender rights, one student leader summed up the grit and the joy of organizing for gender equity:

> Last year I stood before you many times, surrounded by passionate peers, students deeply dedicated to

> improving our community. I was scared that my voice alone couldn't drive change across an entire district, so, once again, I looked to my teachers and staff who have always been by my side. . . . While the national political landscape becomes increasingly uncertain, and frankly terrifying, I find comfort in knowing that [the district] stands firm in its commitment to protecting its students. . . . Let this resolution serve as a reminder: Progress is possible. It is worth the effort. And we can, and we must, do better. −16-year-old nonbinary student

With increasing threats to the health and well-being of transgender people in the United States, this project offers a concrete model of transaffirmative policy change and an example of the courage, hope, and resistance of the transgender student organizers. Beyond its contributions to positive health outcomes, public health policy advocacy can offer an avenue for transgender youth leadership, activism, and joy. AJPH

ABOUT THE AUTHORS

Sonja Mackenzie is with the Department of Public Health at Santa Clara University, Santa Clara, CA. Neha Mann was a student in the Department of Public Health at Santa Clara University at the time of this project. October Hertenstein was a high school student and student activist in Northern California at the time of this project.

CORRESPONDENCE

Correspondence should be sent to Sonja Mackenzie, DrPH, Department of Public Health, Santa Clara University, 500 El Camino Real, Santa Clara, CA 95053 (e-mail: smackenzie@scu.edu). Reprints can be ordered at https://www.ajph.org by clicking the "Reprints" link.

PUBLICATION INFORMATION

Full Citation: Mackenzie S, Mann N, Hertenstein O. Transgender youth health and joy: a model of evidence-based school district policy change to support transgender and nonbinary youth health. *Am J Public Health*. 2026;116(2):210–213.

Acceptance Date: July 30, 2025.

DOI: https://doi.org/10.2105/AJPH.2025.308264

ORCID iDs:
Sonja Mackenzie https://orcid.org/0000-0002-9163-576X

Neha Mann https://orcid.org/0009-0005-6653-7454

October Hertenstein https://orcid.org/0009-0009-7368-9658

CONTRIBUTORS

All coauthors contributed equally to the project. S. Mackenzie led the writing of this article. N. Mann conceptualized Figure 1 and edited the article. O. Hertenstein led the youth organizing and reviewed the article.

CONFLICTS OF INTEREST

There are no conflicts of interest to report on the part of any of the coauthors.

HUMAN PARTICIPANT PROTECTION

No human participant approval was required because this was not a research study.

REFERENCES

1. Trans Legislation Tracker. 2025 anti-trans bills. 2025. Available at: https://translegislation.com. Accessed October 25, 2025.
2. Lee WY, Hobbs JN, Hobaica S, DeChants JP, Price MN, Nath R. State-level anti-transgender laws increase past-year suicide attempts among transgender and non-binary young people in the USA. *Nat Hum Behav*. 2024;8(11):2096–2106. https://doi.org/10.1038/s41562-024-01979-5
3. Summers H, Joe JR. Impact of state legislation on LGBTQIA+ youth in schools. *J LGBTQ Issues Couns*. 2024;18(3):253–266. https://doi.org/10.1080/26924951.2024.2370206
4. The Trevor Project. 2023 US National Survey on the Mental Health of LGBTQ+ Young People. 2023. Available at: https://www.thetrevorproject.org/survey-2023. Accessed October 8, 2025.
5. Price-Feeney M, Green AE, Dorison SH. Impact of bathroom discrimination on mental health among transgender and nonbinary youth. *J Adolesc Health*. 2021;68(6):1142–1147. https://doi.org/10.1016/j.jadohealth.2020.11.001
6. Burson E, Renley BM, Layland EK, et al. Associations between state-level structural stigma and sexual and gender minority youth mental health. *Sex Res Soc Policy*. Published online January 22 2025. https://doi.org/10.1007/s13178-024-01073-5
7. Gabbert L. San Jose parent gets school district to support LGBTQ rights. *San José Spotlight*. August 25, 2023. Available at: https://sanjosespotlight.com/san-jose-parent-gets-school-district-to-support-lgbtq-rights. Accessed February 23, 2025.
8. Rector K, Blume H, Mays M. Right wing targets gender identity; Conservatives wage a well-coordinated, anti-LGBTQ+ culture war in school districts across California. *Los Angeles Times*. October 15, 2023. Available at: https://www.latimes.com/california/story/2023-10-15/how-a-raging-battle-over-lgbtq-issues-in-southern-california-schools-erupted. Accessed February 23, 2025.
9. Abela D, Patlamazoglou L, Lea S. The resistance of transgender and gender expansive people: a scoping review. *Psychol Sex Orientat Gend Divers*. Published online 2024. https://doi.org/10.1037/sgd0000736
10. Equality California Institute: Safe and Supportive Schools Resource Center. Forced outing. Available at: https://safesupportiveschools.org/tag/forced-outing. Accessed October 6, 2025.
11. Lambert D, Velez M. Newsom signs bill to end parental notification policies at schools; opponents say fight is not over. EdSource. Available at: https://edsource.org/2024/newsom-signs-bill-to-end-parental-notification-policies-at-schools-but-opponents-say-its-not-over-yet/715767. Accessed February 28, 2025.
12. Jones C. California bans schools from forcing teachers to "out" LGBTQ students. *CalMatters* December 23, 2024. Available at: http://calmatters.org/education/k-12-education/2024/12/california-forced-outing-lgbtq-new-laws-2025. Accessed February 23, 2025.
13. *California Healthy Kids Survey, 2021–2022: Main Report*. Unified School District. San Francisco, CA: WestEd for the California Department of Education; 2022.
14. Gender Expansive Youth Activists. Press release: School board meeting 03.04.24. *Notion*. March 2024. Available at: https://fizywater-jpg.notion.site/School-Board-Meeting-03-06-24-1b697f60e81f8051a47ccc5cefa56b38#1b697f60e81f8066bb58ef328e5cc360. Accessed March 13, 2025.
15. Herman J, Flores A, O'Neill K. How many adults and youth identify as transgender in the United States? The Williams Institute, UCLA School of Law. 2022. Available at: https://williamsinstitute.law.ucla.edu/publications/trans-adults-united-states. Accessed March 10, 2025.

Sex-Positive HIV Prevention Messages: A Case Study From the Early Years of the Epidemic

Casey W. Adrian, LMSW, Sean G. Massey, PhD, Julia B. Haager, PhD, and Eden Lowinger, LMSW

See also LGBTQ+ Well-Being and Joy, pp. 188–250.

Beginning with the emergence of the HIV/AIDS epidemic in the early 1980s, community-led lesbian, gay, bisexual, and transgender health organizations created prevention materials that affirmed and celebrated gay identity, positing safer sex as a radical method of keeping their communities healthy and liberated past the onset of the virus. Often prioritizing pleasure and featuring erotic imagery, these strengths-based prevention messages implied that community members shared a collective responsibility to care for each other and stop the spread of HIV.

Using archival public health materials from the early HIV/AIDS crisis and data collected through oral history interviews with former members of AIDS service organizations, this article explores the roles that gay liberation, community connectedness, and eroticism played in the first decade of HIV prevention messaging. As a case study, this article highlights the works created by GMHC (formally Gay Men's Health Crisis), New York City's premier AIDS service organization and a global leader in these campaigns.

Lastly, we note similarities between historic examples of sex-positive prevention messaging and those used by community health organizations and practitioners in the 21st century. (*Am J Public Health*. 2026;116(2):214–221. https://doi.org/10.2105/AJPH.2025.308214)

AJPH February 2026, Vol. 116, No. 2

It is April 8, 1982. The inaugural president of Gay Men's Health Crisis (GMHC), Paul Popham, stands onstage at the Paradise Garage, a discotheque in Greenwich Village that caters to a mostly gay clientele. Two hundred people are in attendance for the evening's event: the first fundraiser for GMHC, a new organization established to address the still mysterious "gay cancer" sweeping through communities of men in New York City. An impassioned Popham addresses the audience of lesbian, gay, bisexual, and transgender (LGBT) community members: "We are in the grip of a medical emergency. . . . The finest minds in medicine are on our side, but the problem is still ours. . . . We've got to show the world that we've got more than looks, brains, talent, and money. We've got guts, too. And lots of heart."[1(p62)] Within 5 years of delivering these remarks, Popham would die of complications caused by AIDS.[2]

Popham's speech at the Paradise Garage articulated the strengths-based commitment to the gay community that ran through GMHC's mission and services. By 1992, a decade after this inaugural fundraiser, GMHC positioned itself as a leading resource for medical information, policy and advocacy, social services, legal support, and, notably, culturally responsive prevention education for community members affected by HIV. These health promotion campaigns were created primarily by a workforce of young, LGBT volunteers—people with a vested interest in addressing the unfolding crisis and often with little formal training. Members of GMHC's Prevention Education Department supplemented public health education with knowledge and insights gained from their lived experiences as members of New York City's gay community. David Klotz, a gay man who was 25 and fresh out of university when he was hired as coordinator of prevention services, said of their early work: "We kind of went with our gut—our own knowledge of, you know, public health practice. I mean, I was one of the few that had actually taken courses in public health."[3]

Despite this, many public health professionals, physicians, and health organizations called on GMHC for HIV prevention materials that affirmed and celebrated LGBT identities. Sex educator Patti Britton, who began volunteering in GMHC's Prevention Education Department in 1985 and would later serve in leadership roles for several national sexual and reproductive health organizations, reflected on the agency's instinctual motivations for creating materials that destigmatized gay sex during the height of the crisis:

> Fuck no, we won't go. . . . We've got to do something. And the way to do it is not to terrorize or terrify people. But let's make your use of condoms sexy. Let's talk about how lube can enhance sensation. Let's talk about fucking in new and different ways so that we're not dying from it. And that's appropriate. That was appropriate and it is appropriate.[4]

This article examines sex-positive, strengths-based prevention materials designed by LGBT-led AIDS service organizations (ASOs) in the first decade of the HIV/AIDS epidemic, with a particular focus on GMHC, New York City's premier ASO of the 1980s and 1990s. The authors rely on archival public health documents and organizational records from the time,[5] as well as new collections of archival materials and oral history interviews conducted with former members of GMHC's staff and volunteer workforce, collected by the authors between 2022 and 2024. The research team conducted more than 120 interviews, with participants being sourced through a GMHC alumni Facebook group, informal snowball sampling, and coauthor Sean Massey's personal memory as a former GMHC volunteer and staff person. To complement existing GMHC oral histories available in the New York Public Library, which largely consist of interviews with early members of GMHC leadership, the authors prioritized speaking with former members of the organization's rank-and-file volunteer workforce, including paraprofessionals who were previously involved in the production of these sex-positive prevention campaigns. These new collections of oral histories and archival materials, titled "GMHC Stories: An Oral History Project" and "Sean Massey's Gay Men's Health Crisis Collection," respectively, are in the possession of the Manuscripts, Archives, and Rare Books Division of the New York Public Library and will be available to the public in early 2026.

Lastly, this piece calls attention to examples of sex-positive, LGBT-affirming prevention campaigns created by community-led health organizations and public health practitioners of the 21st century, drawing comparisons between those crafted at the height of the crisis and those still in use today. In examining both historic and contemporary sex-positive prevention materials, we used 3 prominent themes to guide the analysis: gay liberation, community connectedness, and eroticism.

Note that "gay" and "gay and bisexual" were the terminology most often used in the 1980s and 1990s to describe men who had sex with men. As such, the present article uses this terminology to describe the population. The authors acknowledge that this language may not be inclusive of all men who have sex with men. The authors use "LGBT" (lesbian, gay, bisexual, transgender) to describe a broad community of sexually marginalized people, acknowledging that this acronym was not widespread in 1980s and 1990s New York City, while also being mindful of the contributions of lesbians and transgender people in the history of AIDS service work.

GAY LIBERATION

Before the outbreak of the HIV/AIDS epidemic, many LGBT people in major coastal cities of the United States experienced the 1970s as a period of relative liberation, brought on by the increasingly militant homophile movement of the midcentury; the works of progressive scientists (e.g., Alfred Kinsey and Evelyn Hooker), which activists called on to depathologize homosexuality; and spontaneous demonstrations against police harassment and suppression, largely spearheaded by transgender women of color, such as the respective uprisings at Compton's Cafeteria in the summer of 1966 and the Stonewall Inn in the summer of 1969.[6,7] In cities such as New York City and San Francisco, California, this often meant that stigmatized behaviors and identities were becoming more visible. Especially for gay and bisexual men, this included the increasing visibility of a culture that was created and validated through sex. Tim Pinckney, a playwright who formerly volunteered to facilitate GMHC's safer sex workshops, reflected on this pre-AIDS period of LGBT life in New York City:

> The 70s were a very active time. It was a decade of sexual awakening after Stonewall. . . . [Gay men] were finding themselves and expressing themselves. And you started seeing they were more vivid. There was a visibility. And a lot of ways that gay men expressed themselves was through sex. And it was everywhere—and it was rampant. . . . I came in at the tail end of that. I remember sex before condoms.[8]

For gay men who had been raised amid the Lavender Scare and related moral panics of previous decades, acts of unrestricted sex were often seen as

AJPH February 2026, Vol. 116, No. 2

a liberatory reaction to the discriminatory social and political environments of their youths.[6,7]

By the late 1970s, breakouts of hepatitis B and other sexually transmitted infections became visible in coastal communities of gay and bisexual men; as a result, many of these men were called to participate in the clinical trials of the hepatitis B vaccine.[9] James Holmes, a gay man who formerly volunteered in GMHC's Prevention Education Department, recalled his participation in these clinical trials of the 1970s: "They engaged the gay community [in clinical trials of the hepatitis B vaccine] because there was very high infection rates, but they also found that gay men were very compliant. They showed up, they participated, they didn't drop out."[10] Thus, while gay and bisexual men made strides toward depathologizing their sexualities during the 1970s,[11,12] the decade simultaneously resulted in the medicalization of their bodies, priming these young men to think about their health as they likely had not done before.

Beginning in September of 1979, this uptick in sexually transmitted infections prompted the San Francisco–based National Coalition and Bay Area Physicians for Human Rights, organizations of LGBT and LGBT-allied physicians and health professionals, to create intentionally nonjudgmental medical guidelines to prevent the spread of sexually transmitted infections among gay men. In the years to follow, the Sisters of Perpetual Indulgence (a troupe of drag queen nuns with names like Sister Florence Nightmare and Sister Roz Erection) translated this medical information into plain and accessible language that would appeal to members of the community.[13] Such actions taken by LGBT-led activist groups and health organizations demonstrate pre-epidemic examples of outreach materials embedded with the camp and liberatory spirit of increasingly visible LGBT communities.

In July of 1981, when a short piece about a "Rare Cancer Seen in 41 Homosexuals" was published on page 20 of the *New York Times*,[14] a crisis began materializing. The initial response from New York's LGBT community, however, demonstrated a reluctance to surrender their ongoing sexual liberation. The first-ever report on what would later be known as AIDS, published in the gay-led *New York Native* on May 18, 1981 (3 weeks before the coverage by the *New York Times*), ran under the headline "Disease Rumors Largely Unfounded," an instance of the community's knee-jerk refusal to have their sex lives moralized into the new decade.[15] By the end of the year, a group of 80 people, largely gay men who were diversely involved in the ongoing gay liberation movement, met in Larry Kramer's Greenwich Village living room to discuss the mysterious disease affecting their community; a few months later, 6 of these men formed GMHC.

Conflicts emerged among early GMHC leadership regarding the most effective model of health promotion. Before the identification of HIV, incorrect theories of transmission abounded within LGBT communities.[16] Though the virus remained unidentified until May of 1983, it soon became clear that sexual transmission was at least partially responsible for its spread. Some early members of the organization advocated abstinence as the only method of prevention. Promoters of abstinence-oriented prevention included Kramer, a cofounder of GMHC. In Kramer's largely autobiographical play, *The Normal Heart*, the protagonist faces repeated backlash when he advocates for gay men to "cool it" and stop having sex, eventually contributing to his separation from the organization.[17] Others within GMHC, however, understood that gay and bisexual men were unlikely to commit to prevention strategies that threatened to upend the sexual liberation of the previous decade. Holmes recalled of this theoretical approach:

> So there's a 10 year period [before AIDS], during which gay men were sort of breaking out of this very fear-based thing. . . . And gay men typically did—still do—feel very guilty about their practices. So [our sex-positive prevention campaigns were] a way to counter that, saying that we can't get people to change their behavior if they're afraid. . . . Many of us realized that gay men were not going to stop having sex. We needed to figure out a way that they could have sex but do it safely.[10]

COMMUNITY CONNECTEDNESS

To achieve the goal outlined by Holmes, GMHC's Prevention Education Department was tasked with devising outreach materials that uplifted the gay community while urging its members to reconsider their largely unrestricted sexual practices. While much was still unknown about the epidemiology or medical realities of AIDS, one of GMHC's earliest interventions involved promoting monogamous relationships between men. In GMHC's first newsletter, sociologist Martin Levine offered monogamous relationships not as a setback, but as an intimate configuration that could promote both personal well-being and community connectedness:

> With fast tricks 'out,' wedding bands are 'in'; men are coupling off, and lovers are popping up all over town.

> Even veterans of countless one-night stands are giving dating a go. This switch in styles isn't necessarily a bad thing. It could be a positive growth experience. . . . All is not gloom and despair. This challenge gives us the opportunity to prove that we are more than a community of men who fuck each other. We can show ourselves and the world that we are a community of men who love each other. In this crisis, we are family, and we have the talent, money and concern to take care of one another.[18(pp15–16)]

In a similar sentiment, LGBT activists Richard Berkowitz and Michael Callen, in collaboration with gay physician Joseph Sonnabend, published *How to Have Sex in an Epidemic* in 1983, the first sex-positive set of medical guidelines to come out of New York's gay male community. Promoting altruism and closeness between men, both within and outside of monogamous relationships, the authors write: "If you love the person you are fucking with—even for one night—you will not want to make them sick. Maybe affection is our best protection."[19(p39)] Soon, an international audience of gay men, gay-allied physicians, health professionals, and librarians wrote to the authors for copies of these guidelines, including members of the GMHC workforce.[20]

Calling on this sentiment, GMHC's earliest workshops were aimed at providing gay and bisexual men with skills for building compassionate, altruistic relationships that extended beyond casual sex. In November 1985, GMHC held "Close Encounters (of the Best Kind)," a series of 3 workshops, each lasting 2 hours and followed by a community social event. These workshops empowered men to see themselves as part of a larger community with a shared responsibility and capacity to love. Sessions included the aptly titled "Changing the Way You Think About Yourself and Others" ("Developing and maintaining self-esteem in the face of crisis") and "Dating 101" ("What a date is, how to choose a partner, general issues around dating").[21] The third and final workshop in the series, "Eroticizing Healthy Sex," sought to teach participants "how to introduce the concept of healthy sex to your partner" and "how to make [safer sex] fun and hot."[21] In the years to come, this final theme became a major focus of GMHC's prevention messaging: making safer sex attractive and enticing for LGBT people.

EROTICISM

As condoms became increasingly recognized as an effective method of preventing HIV transmission through sex, GMHC made a concerted effort to create prevention materials that promoted their use within the gay male community. Until the mid-1980s, however, condoms had been advertised near-exclusively to heterosexual people, primarily as a form of contraception and, when necessary, as a method of preventing sexually transmitted infections. Because of their association with procreative sex, few gay men saw condoms as being relevant to their lives or sexual practices, more often ascribing this form of protection as something heterosexual in nature.[22] As Klotz reflected:

> Telling gay men, who had been completely uninhibited, that suddenly they're [going to] have to start using condoms for the rest of their lives—it was a difficult message. I mean, in the '70s and early '80s, when gay men came out, one of the great things about sex as a gay man is he didn't have to worry about getting somebody pregnant. So why wear condoms?[3]

GMHC responded to this by creating prevention materials that eroticized condom use for LGBT audiences. One landmark example of this was their *Safer Sex Condom Guide for Men and Women* (Figure 1), published in 1987, which Britton (who served as the hand model for this piece of prevention material) called the "first [sexually explicit] brochure ever made, ever designed and printed, on the safer use of condoms."[4] The guide used sexually explicit photographs to demonstrate the proper use of a condom, from opening the foil to removal after ejaculation. An image of 2 naked men in an embrace is stretched across the centerfold, aimed at making condoms feel sexy and relevant in the lives of gay men. The guide encouraged readers to experiment with different condoms before settling on the ones that they prefer ("When you buy other things, don't you shop around?") and offered creative ideas for making condom use into a form of foreplay ("Use your imagination. Think of new and fun ways to play with rubbers. Think of new ways to put them on.").[23]

The condom guide is not the only example of provocative and sexually explicit imagery in GMHC's prevention materials. For a brief list, one could look at GMHC's *Safer Sex Comix*, a series of 7 black-and-white cartoon books created between 1986 and 1987, each filled with erotic stories of men negotiating the creative use of condoms and nonpenetrative sex acts. GMHC's "Young, Hot, Safe" advertisements, posted in New York City subway cars after an uptick in adolescent HIV infections in the early to mid-1990s, featured images of young, racially diverse,

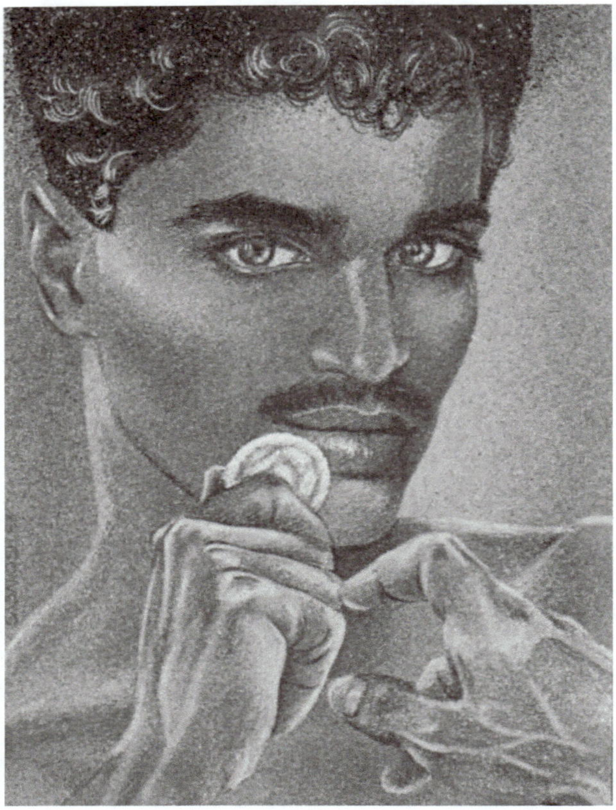

FIGURE 1— Gay Men's Health Crisis's Safer Sex Condom Guide for Men and Women, Page 1

Note. This brochure is a part of the Sean Massey's Gay Men's Health Crisis Collection in the New York Public Library's Manuscripts, Archives and Rare Books Division, available in early 2026.[23]

same-sex couples nuzzling and kissing while holding condoms and other protective devices. Their *Safer Sex Shorts*, produced by Jean Carlomusto and Greg Bordowitz, were pornographic videos in which people had sex using various forms of protection, filmed with the intention of being played at bathhouses and other public sex venues.

Of note, GMHC's explicit and sex-positive materials were not without controversies, both from members of the LGBT community and from oppressive political actors on the outside. As AIDS became more visible in women and people of color in the late 1980s and 1990s, critics both within and external to the organization condemned GMHC for attempting to adapt their "gay model" of prevention (eroticizing condom use through gay male pornography and vernacular) to reach other demographics of people at risk, such as those on the "downlow"—men, especially those of color, who identified as heterosexual and had sex with other men.[24,25]

Other controversies played out in a more public manner. Religious subway passengers expressed opposition to the "Young, Hot, Safe" posters being shown in train cars, insisting that such displays of healthy youth sexuality were forms of "indoctrination, to re-educate our children to reject their religious upbringing in favor of liberal, secularist and moral relativism."[26] This resulted in a screaming match at a City Council meeting between AIDS activists in favor of the prevention campaign and religious leaders who opposed the effort.[27] In another example, on October 14, 1987, Senator Jesse Helms of North Carolina brought a copy of *GMHC Safer Sex Comix #6* to the Senate floor (Figure 2). In this small booklet of cartoons, the fictional "all-star jock-stud Ed" and "dark pumpboy Julio" make an erotic show of unrolling condoms and practicing safer sex,[28] part of GMHC's effort to demonstrate how protection can enhance pleasure between men. Holding the comic book in his hand, Helms proclaimed to Ronald Reagan and his fellow senators:

> Mr. President, this Senator is not a goody-goody two-shoes. I have lived a long time. I have seen a lot of things. . . . But every Christian, religious, moral ethic within me cries out to do something. It is embarrassing to stand on the Senate floor and talk about the details of this travesty. . . . I will not consume the Senate's time reading the details of this revolting project. But, Mr. President, you know those little bags they have on airplanes when it gets bumpy. If I were to read the sickening details to you, Mr. President, you would need one.[29(p27 753)]

With this, Senator Helms successfully passed an amendment spending bill by a vote of 94 to 2, prohibiting federal funds from being used to provide AIDS education, information, or prevention materials that promoted, encouraged, or condoned homosexual sexual activities. With federal funds making up roughly 15% of their operating budget at the time, this legislation threatened to completely undermine GMHC's strategy of sex-positive and identity-affirming prevention for LGBT people.

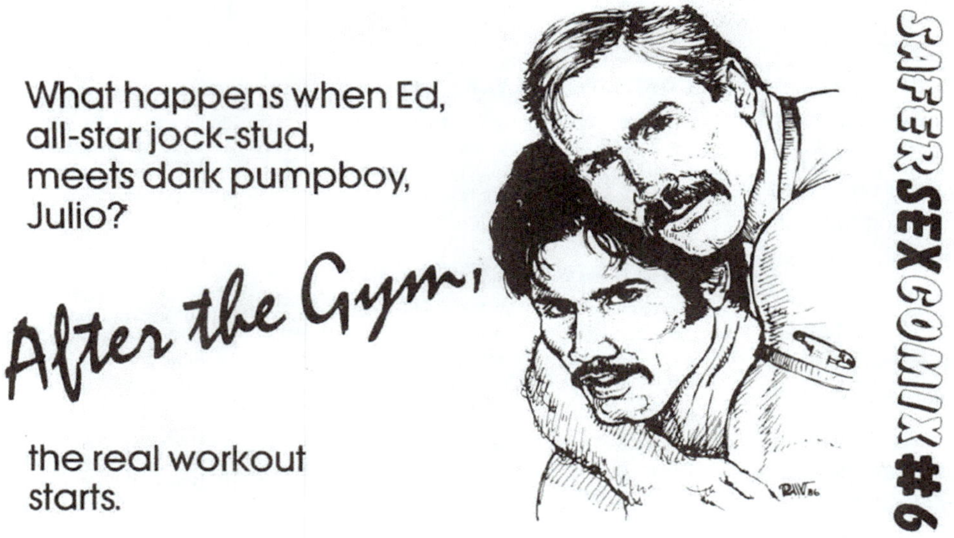

FIGURE 2— Gay Men's Health Crisis's Safer Sex Comix #6, Front Cover

Note. Senator Jesse Helms held this pamphlet on the floor of the Senate on October 14, 1987. This is a part of the Sean Massey's Gay Men's Health Crisis Collection in the New York Public Library's Manuscripts, Archives and Rare Books Division, available in early 2026.[28]

AJPH February 2026, Vol. 116, No. 2

In situations such as these, however, GMHC called on their large and stalwart base of supporters, successfully using their position as a political scapegoat to catalyze fundraising efforts, as most prospective donors were similarly affected by displays of structural homophobia. Katharine DeShaw, who served as director of GMHC's Development Department between 1988 and 1991, shared: "So, in other words, if you got [government dollars], great. But don't count on them. What we knew we could count on was private philanthropy."[30] DeShaw's approach to fundraising at GMHC speaks of course to the financial means of the agency's earliest clientele, workforce, and broader social network, but also to the solidarity and resilience throughout the community at the time. In instances such as these, many LGBT people rallied around sex-positive and identity-affirming HIV prevention, refusing to submit not only to the virus itself but also to an oppressive political landscape that was indifferent to their survival.

LASTING LEGACIES

With their sexual freedom, collective identities, and very lives at stake, GMHC and other ASOs of the early HIV/AIDS epidemic committed themselves to designing creative, strengths-based approaches to sexual health promotion. These safer-sex campaigns sought to sustain gay liberation past the outbreak of the virus, pushing LGBT people to reimagine sex, their relationships, and what it meant to be intimate with each other. Into the second and third decades of the epidemic, other organizations went on to create similarly erotic materials, aimed at promoting altruism between gay men—such as one poster from the AIDS Action Committee of Massachusetts, featuring a photo of 2 young men engaged in anal sex, which encouraged men to wear condoms by saying: "Is he just a piece of meat? Do you care about him at all? . . . If he can't look out for himself, then you'll have to."[31] As the epidemic continued through the 1990s and 2000s, GMHC pivoted to create prevention messages aimed at addressing safer sex fatigue among gay and bisexual men—such as their Staying Negative campaign, which validated those who were burnt out by a decade of constant health anxiety while also using destigmatizing language to encourage continued harm reduction. Above a telephone number for the GMHC hotline, one 1995 pamphlet read: "By talking about the sex you are having, what it means to you, and what it may cost you, it is possible to make partying—and sex—safer."[32]

Into the 21st century, many public health practitioners continue to utilize themes of liberation, community connectedness, and eroticism to promote safer sexual behaviors and attempt to circumvent the negative consequences of stigma. One may look, for instance, at the "We Prevent" intervention for young men who have sex with men or the "2GETHER" intervention for same-sex male couples,[33,34] each reminiscent of attempts to build relationship skills and foster closeness between men during the early crisis. Other examples include the Chicago-based "PrEP4Love" campaign, a sex-positive effort that used intimate and erotic photographs of same-sex couples to market preexposure prophylaxis uptake,[35,36] or materials created by the National Coalition for Sexual Health at the outbreak of the mpox virus in the United States, which feature images of men kissing and embracing with captions that frame sexual health services as means of enhancing pleasure and intimacy; for instance, one included the caption: "Want to worry less and enjoy sex more? Get the mpox vaccine."[37] Far from an exhaustive list, these examples demonstrate how contemporary community health organizations equip sex-positivity and identity-affirmation in their messaging—social marketing that posits prevention as a method of sustaining liberation, building community, and enhancing pleasure.

There are opportunities for future research studies to explore and detail the ways in which these materials may promote healthier sexual behaviors while simultaneously fostering pride, solidarity, and closeness among LGBT people. These stories demonstrate that, even in the face of oppressive governmental forces and unrelenting hardship, LGBT health advocates are able to reach into the strengths of their communities, rally around each other, and maintain the momentum of progress that has been made. AJPH

ABOUT THE AUTHORS

Casey W. Adrian is with the Bronfenbrenner Center for Translational Research, Cornell University, Ithaca, NY. Sean G. Massey is with the Women, Gender & Sexuality Studies Program, Binghamton University, Binghamton, NY. Julia B. Haager is with the Department of History, Western Carolina University, Cullowhee, NC. Eden Lowinger was with the Department of Social Work, Binghamton University, Binghamton, NY, at the time of this study.

CORRESPONDENCE

Correspondence should be sent to Casey W. Adrian, LMSW, 1201 Martha Van Rensselaer Hall, Cornell University, Ithaca, NY 14853 (e-mail: cwa39@cornell.edu). Reprints can be ordered at https://www.ajph.org by clicking the "Reprints" link.

PUBLICATION INFORMATION

Full Citation: Adrian CW, Massey SG, Haager JB, Lowinger E. Sex-positive HIV prevention messages: a case study from the early years of the epidemic. *Am J Public Health*. 2026;116(2):214–221.

Acceptance Date: June 8, 2025.

DOI: https://doi.org/10.2105/AJPH.2025.308214

ORCID iDs:

Casey W. Adrian https://orcid.org/0009-0008-4470-6634

Sean G. Massey https://orcid.org/0000-0001-5984-7116

Julia B. Haager https://orcid.org/0000-0002-0655-566X

Eden Lowinger https://orcid.org/0009-0008-7949-3026

CONTRIBUTORS

C. W. Adrian conceptualized and led the writing of this piece. S. G. Massey and J. B. Haager co-led the archival and oral history projects from which these sources were pulled and contributed to writing and analysis for this essay. E. Lowinger provided crucial insights throughout each step of the research and writing processes.

ACKNOWLEDGMENTS

The authors would like to acknowledge the Manuscripts, Archives and Rare Books Division of the New York Public Library for accepting these oral history interviews and archival materials into their collections, each of which will be made available to the public in early 2026. Special thanks to the library's Julie Golia, PhD, for her countless contributions to the process. The authors also acknowledge the Gay Men's Health Crisis records collection that was donated to the New York Public Library in the mid-1990s. Lastly, the authors would like to recognize the 120 former members of Gay Men's Health Crisis's workforce who contributed their voices, stories, and personal collections to these oral history and archival projects.

CONFLICTS OF INTEREST

The authors have no conflicts of interest to disclose.

HUMAN PARTICIPANT PROTECTION

The authors' institutions did not require institutional review board approval for these interviews, as they were collected as oral histories.

REFERENCES

1. VerMeulen M. The gay plague: A mysterious immune disorder is spreading like wildfire. *New York Magazine*. May 31, 1982:15(22):52–62.
2. Rosenthal A. Paul Popham, 45, a founder of AIDS organization, dies. *New York Times*. May 8, 1987:D17.
3. Klotz D, interviewed by Massey SG, Haager JB, Goldstein C, Lowinger E. *GMHC Stories: An Oral History Project*. 2022. Forthcoming at: New York Public Library, New York, NY.
4. Britton P, interviewed by Massey SG, Haager JB, Adrian CW, Goldstein C, Pergel D. *GMHC Stories: An Oral History Project*. 2022. Forthcoming at: New York Public Library, New York, NY.
5. Gay Men's Health Crisis records. Manuscripts and Archives Division, The New York Public Library. Available at: https://archives.nypl.org/mss/1126#overview. Accessed January 15, 2025.
6. D'Emilio J. Dreams deferred: The birth and betrayal of America's first Gay Liberation Movement. In: *Making Trouble: Essays on Gay History, Politics, and the University*. New York, NY: Routledge; 1992:17–56.
7. D'Emilio J. *Sexual Politics, Sexual Communities: The Making of a Homosexual Minority in the United States, 1940–1970*. Chicago, IL: The University of Chicago Press; 1998.
8. Pinckney T, interviewed by Massey SG, Haager JB, Adrian CW, Goldstein C, Pergel D. *GMHC Stories: An Oral History Project*. 2022. Forthcoming at: New York Public Library, New York, NY.
9. Hessol NA, Lifson AR, O'Malley PM, Doll LS, Jaffe HW, Rutherford GW. Prevalence, incidence, and progression of human immunodeficiency virus infection in homosexual and bisexual men in hepatitis B vaccine trials, 1978–1988. *Am J Epidemiol*. 1989;130(6):1167–1175. https://doi.org/10.1093/oxfordjournals.aje.a115445
10. Holmes J, interviewed by Massey SG, Haager JB, Adrian CW, Goldstein C, Morea S, Pergel D. 2022. *GMHC Stories: An Oral History Project*. Forthcoming at: New York Public Library, New York, NY.
11. Lewis AJ. "We are certain of our own insanity": antipsychiatry and the Gay Liberation Movement, 1968–1980. *J Hist Sex*. 2016;25(1):83–113. https://doi.org/10.7560/jhs25104
12. Drescher J. Out of *DSM*: depathologizing homosexuality. *Behav Sci (Basel)*. 2015;5(4):565–575. https://doi.org/10.3390/bs5040565
13. Blair TR. Safe sex in the 1970s: community practitioners on the eve of AIDS. *Am J Public Health*. 2017;107(6):872–879. https://doi.org/10.2105/ajph.2017.303704
14. Altman L. Rare cancer seen in 41 homosexuals. *New York Times*. July 3, 1981:A20.
15. Mass L. Disease rumors largely unfounded. *New York Native*. May 18, 1981:A7.
16. Nattrass N. *The AIDS Conspiracy: Science Fights Back*. New York, NY: Columbia University Press; 2013.
17. Kramer L. *The Normal Heart*. London, UK: Nick Hern Books; 1985.
18. Levine M. Fearing fear itself. In: *GMHC Newsletter 1*. 1982. Gay Men's Health Crisis records. Located at: New York Public Library, New York, NY.
19. Berkowitz R, Callen M, Sonnabend J. *How to Have Sex in an Epidemic: One Approach*. Dworkin R, ed. New York, NY: News From the Front Publications; 1983.

20. Lloyd-Jones J. Who was reading "How to have sex in an epidemic"? Library, Archive & Open Research Services Blog. December 12, 2014. Available at: https://blogs.lshtm.ac.uk/library/2014/12/12/reading-sex-epidemic. Accessed January 15, 2025.
21. Gay Men's Health Crisis. Crisis management partner team #1 meeting minutes. October 9, 1985. *Sean Massey's Gay Men's Health Crisis Collection*. Forthcoming at: New York Public Library, New York, NY.
22. Brier J. Marketing safer sex: the politics of sexuality, race, and class in San Francisco. In: *Infectious Ideas: US Political Responses to the AIDS Crisis.* Chapel Hill, NC: University of North Carolina Press; 2009:45–77.
23. GMHC Publications. The safer sex condom guide for men and women. 1987. *Sean Massey's Gay Men's Health Crisis Collection*. Forthcoming at: New York Public Library, New York, NY.
24. Robinson C. 53% is no minority. In: *The Volunteer.* 3:7. 1986. *Sean Massey's Gay Men's Health Crisis Collection*. Forthcoming at: New York Public Library, New York, NY.
25. Wright GP, interviewed by Massey SG, Haager J, Lowinger E, Morea S, Pergel D. 2022. *GMHC Stories: An Oral History Project.* Forthcoming at: New York Public Library, New York, NY.
26. Kerrison R. Sleazy AIDS ads take the gay train. *New York Post*. January 19, 1994; Section 1:2, 16.
27. Lugliani G. Memorandum to all GMHC staff. January 31, 1994. *Sean Massey's Gay Men's Health Crisis Collection*. Forthcoming at: New York Public Library, New York, NY.
28. GMHC Publications. *GMHC Safer Sex Comix #6*. 1986. *Sean Massey's Gay Men's Health Crisis Collection*. Forthcoming at: New York Public Library, New York, NY.
29. Congressional Record. 100th Cong, 1st Sess. Vol 133, pt 20. Senate. October 14, 1987:27747–27844.
30. DeShaw K, interviewed by Massey SG, Haager JB, Adrian CW, Pergel D. 2022. *GMHC Stories: An Oral History Project.* Forthcoming at: New York Public Library, New York, NY.
31. AIDS Action Committee of Massachusetts, Better World Advertising. Is He Just a Piece of Meat?: Do You Care about Him at All?: Making Contact. Available at: http://resource.nlm.nih.gov/101717734?_gl=1*1mgq41l*_ga*MTI2MTI5ODc0OC4xNzE3NzgxNTc0*_ga_7147EPK006*czE3NDcyNDQ4NDMkbzIkZzEkdDE3NDcyNDU3NTEkajAkbDAkaDA. Accessed January 15, 2025.
32. GMHC Publications. *Staying Negative – It's Not Automatic*. 1995. *Sean Massey's Gay Men's Health Crisis Collection*. Forthcoming at: New York Public Library, New York, NY.
33. Gamarel KE, Darbes LA, Hightow-Weidman L, Sullivan P, Stephenson R. The development and testing of a relationship skills intervention to improve HIV prevention uptake among young gay, bisexual, and other men who have sex with men and their primary partners (We Prevent): protocol for a randomized controlled trial. *JMIR Res Protoc.* 2019;8(1):e10370. https://doi.org/10.2196/10370
34. Newcomb ME, Macapagal KR, Feinstein BA, Bettin E, Swann G, Whitton SW. Integrating HIV prevention and relationship education for young same-sex male couples: a pilot trial of the 2GETHER Intervention. *AIDS Behav.* 2017;21(8):2464–2478. https://doi.org/10.1007/s10461-017-1674-0
35. Phillips G, Raman AB, Felt D, et al. PrEP4Love: the role of messaging and prevention advocacy in PrEP attitudes, perceptions, and uptake among YMSM and transgender women. *J Acquir Immune Defic Syndr.* 2020;83(5):450–456. https://doi.org/10.1097/qai.0000000000002297
36. Keene LC, Dehlin JM, Pickett J, et al. #PrEP4Love: success and stigma following release of the first sex-positive PrEP public health campaign. *Cult Health Sex.* 2021;23(3):397–413. https://doi.org/10.1080/13691058.2020.1715482
37. Altarum Institute. Mpox vaccine promotion materials toolkit. 2024. Available at: https://www.nationalcoalitionforsexualhealth.org/tools/for-healthcare-providers/mpox-toolkit. Accessed January 15, 2025.

Unconventional Resilience: Necessary Social Identity Management Among Asylum-Seeking Sexual and Gender-Diverse Survival Migrants

David Chinyeaka Agor, DNP, Chioma Nnaji, MPH, MEd, Carmen Alvarez, MSN, PhD, Jose Bauermeister, PhD, MPH, and Steven Meanley, PhD, MPH

See also LGBTQ+ Well-Being and Joy, pp. 188–250.

Sexual and gender-diverse (SGD) survival migrants face unique challenges navigating multilevel stigma across migratory phases while seeking asylum in the United States. This analytic essay extends Ungar's social-ecological conceptualization of resilience to understand how SGD survival migrants strategically manage their identities within traumatogenic processes to progress from survival to flourishing.

We examine 2 critical migration-related stressors: the social visibility dilemma and intersectional concealability. The social visibility dilemma emerges from US asylum requirements mandating visible SGD identity demonstration, creating paradoxical pressures for individuals conditioned to conceal their identities in high-stigma environments and avoid associated stigma for loved ones in their countries of origin. Intersectional concealability refers to how multiple stigmatized identities perceived by others may launch stigma cascades operating through mechanisms of contextual believability and perception-based cascades.

Resilience among SGD survival migrants reflects atypical, culturally relative strategies that challenge Global Northern paradigms of identity coherence. Public health practitioners and policymakers must recognize that apparent inconsistency often represents sophisticated adaptation within constrained environments. Recommendations include trauma-informed mental health care, peer support networks, asylum process reforms protecting confidentiality, and validation of diverse identity expressions beyond Global Northern visibility norms. (*Am J Public Health*. 2026;116(2):222–228. https://doi.org/10.2105/AJPH.2025.308337)

AJPH February 2026, Vol. 116, No. 2

Sexual and gender-diverse (SGD) individuals, including those who identify as lesbian, gay, bisexual, transgender, queer, and other nonheterosexual and gender-expansive identities, face profound challenges to their safety, well-being, and human dignity across the globe.[1–3] In 69 countries (mainly in the Global South), same-sex relationships and gender-diverse identity and expression remain criminalized, with 11 of these countries imposing the death penalty.[3,4] The criminalization of these lived experiences reflects state-sanctioned structural stigma and creates hostile environments where SGD individuals face increased risk of interpersonal stigma and social stress. Hostile environments can be evaluated via scores (i.e., scores below 5 points) on the Global Acceptance Index (e.g., scores for Ethiopia, Indonesia, Russia, and Haiti are 1.63, 2.70, 3.28, and 3.32, respectively).[5]

State-sanctioned structural stigma cascades across social ecological levels, with SGD individuals being discriminated against by mainstream society, viewed as second-class citizens, and victimized in ways that severely constrain their access to vital social determinants of health.[6–8] At the interpersonal level, state-sanctioned structural stigma may enable or promote co-occurring experiences of victimization (i.e., polyvictimization) such as corrective rape, intimate partner violence, human trafficking, physical assault, psychological torture, and chronic harassment.[2–4]

As a result of the persecution experienced by SGD individuals on the basis of their perceived or disclosed SGD identity, individuals are often forced to pursue "survival migration."[1,9] Survival migration is a strategy of pursuing safer, more affirming environments that provide access to fundamental human rights, including the right to life, authentic self-expression, and potential for flourishing.[9,10] Furthermore, throughout the migratory phases (premigration, migration, and postmigration),[3,4] strategic identity navigation is essential for the survival and resilience of SGD survival migrants.[9,11,12] For instance, SGD survival migrants must identify and monitor when it is safe to disclose their SGD identity as they navigate seeking migration-related resources and support.[6,13] The fear, anticipation, and perceived consequences of multilevel stigma attributed to being an SGD survival migrant pose heightened risks for polyvictimization and psychological distress, including anxiety, depression, posttraumatic stress disorder, and suicidality.[4,6]

Beyond their own multilevel experiences of stigma, SGD survival migrants also experience a significant burden resulting from the constant vigilance required to shield loved ones from the damaging effects of associated stigma (also referred to as courtesy stigma).[3,14] Associated stigma occurs when friends or family members of SGD migrants experience persecution, polyvictimization, and marginalization simply for being associated with an SGD person.[6,8] Associated stigma poses a threat to the safety and well-being of family members who continue to reside in SGD survival migrants' country of origin or other SGD high-structural-stigma environments[14,15] and typifies the transnationalism of SGD multilevel stigma.[16] Furthermore, associated stigma elicits added stress throughout the migratory phases for SGD survival migrants, creating a high perceived need for strategic SGD identity management.[14,15]

Until recently, the United States was long regarded as a global leader in considering asylum applications from SGD survival migrants arriving from countries with state-sanctioned hostile environments, both by establishing precedent-setting legal protections and by granting asylum at comparatively higher rates than many peer nations. Unlike other migrant populations where a healthy migrant paradox has been observed[4,17] (e.g., the "Latino paradox," in which Latino immigrants arrive with better health profiles than US-born Latinos despite socioeconomic disadvantages), current data suggest that SGD survival migrants arrive in the United States with a higher burden of psychological distress than both US-born SGD individuals and other migrants. This reversal underscores how hostile state-sanctioned environments and anticipatory stigma before migration produce a health burden that persists across borders, neutralizing the protective effects typically associated with the migration process. Yet, paradoxically, many adapt, flourish, and thrive, demonstrating remarkable resilience that emerges within these traumatogenic contexts.[12,18,19]

Although understanding SGD survival migrants' experiences through trauma-focused frameworks is vital for documenting these harms, this approach undermines the multilevel creative strategies and assets that migrants marshal to navigate intersectional stigma.[11,12] How SGD survival migrants operate within sociopolitical constraints, where survival and thriving depend on individual navigation skills and available multilevel assets, remains underexplored.[4,11] Crucially, highlighting their resilience does not diminish the reality of hostile environments; rather, it underscores the paradox that resilience itself is a byproduct and necessity resulting from surviving structural hostility.

We acknowledge critical perspectives that caution against framing resilience as uniformly positive. Some scholars argue that resilience may itself be an adverse event, insofar as it normalizes the expectation that marginalized groups must adapt to systemic violence rather than compelling structural change.[18–20] For SGD survival migrants, resilience is both empowering and burdensome: it reflects extraordinary adaptive strategies, yet it also represents the "scar tissue" of traumatogenic environments. Here we seek to hold this paradox in view; we recognize resilience as a necessary survival strategy while refusing to romanticize it or obscure the systemic forces that make such resilience necessary.

CONCEPTUALIZATION OF RESILIENCE FOR SURVIVAL MIGRANTS

Guided by the principles outlined in Ungar's social-ecological conceptualization of resilience, we aim to raise awareness and unpack understudied multilevel stigma and atypical resilience employed by SGD survival migrants in the Global North, namely, the social visibility dilemma and intersectional identity concealability. Ungar's social-ecological conceptualization of resilience provides a robust framework for understanding the complex navigation

AJPH February 2026, Vol. 116, No. 2

strategies employed by SGD survival migrants.[21,22]

The social-ecological conceptualization of resilience recognizes it as a bidirectional relationship between an individual and the environment—the capacity of individuals and their environments to interact in ways that promote well-being and buffer against risk—based on the principles of decentrality, atypicality, and cultural relativity.[21,22] Decentrality is the notion that resilience is not just an individual asset but encompasses the broader environment and systems that support individuals in overcoming negative circumstances. It decenters individuals (i.e., SGD survival migrants) and accentuates structures and policies that create opportunities for accessing needed support. In the context of SGD survival migrants, legal protections, asylum access, and antidiscrimination policies are structural assets.

Atypicality is a principle that suggests resilience does not manifest identically across individuals and cultures.[21,22] Individuals demonstrate resilience in diverse, sometimes seemingly unconventional ways that serve as an adaptive function of their lived experiences. Coping mechanisms often labeled as maladaptive or harmful by dominant Global North perspectives may actually be rational responses to high-structural-stigma environments.[11,12,22] In other words, resilience strategies do not always appear outwardly positive. For example, studies show that concealment is maladaptive for SGD people in the lower structural environment and are associated with psychological distress. However, concealment is physical and neuroprotective, mitigates stigma cascades and escape, and limits awareness of multilevel stigma and polyvictimization for SGD populations in higher-structural-stigma environments.[23,24] SGD survival migrants may engage in atypical coping behaviors across the migratory phases that serve to facilitate physical and emotional self-preservation.[11,12]

Cultural relativity acknowledges that adaptive behaviors vary across cultural contexts, illuminating the challenges SGD survival migrants face when navigating between divergent cultural frameworks of identity.[21,22] Cultural relativity accentuates equifinality of resilience, which is defined as multiple pathways that lead to resilience; however, it is prioritized by cultural and individual values and needs. For example, a successful asylum application typifies equifinality for SGD survival migrants.[11,12] Strategies that promote resilience in one cultural context may not be relevant or effective in another. Cultural values, norms, and resources shape how resilience is expressed and supported.

THE SOCIAL VISIBILITY DILEMMA

As part of this analytic essay, we expand on Ungar's framework to include stressors specific to the migratory phase among SGD survival migrants. Figure 1 provides a conceptual framework depicting how the social visibility dilemma and intersectional concealability may expand our understanding of atypical multilevel resilience processes among SGD survival migrants. These experiences are critical to an understanding of SGD survival migrants' resilience and trajectories toward thriving and flourishing in the postmigration phase.

For SGD survival migrants, identities related to sexual orientation, gender identity, immigration status, and race/ethnicity create unique vulnerability patterns at their intersections.[2,4] These identity dimensions vary in visibility across different contexts, creating nuanced experiences of stigmatization that cannot be reduced to single categories. Although the visibility and credibility of these intersecting minoritized identities are not inherently pathological, they can trigger cascades of stigmatization leading to discrimination and restricted access to resources essential for optimal health, well-being, and quality of life.[2,6]

When seeking asylum, SGD survival migrants often perceive a need to balance multiple individual, social, and cultural priorities, put simply their equifinality: securing legal status, maintaining credibility, preserving SGD community connections, and protecting family and friends from associated stigma.[2,15] Balancing these priorities often creates social challenges for SGD survival migrants as they seek and are granted asylum. The social visibility dilemma represents a critical paradox for SGD survival migrants navigating the US asylum system.[2] It encompasses individuals' strategic navigation of identity disclosures to meet the legal requirements for being granted asylum.

US asylum policies mandate that SGD asylum seekers demonstrate SGD community membership according to the "social visibility clause,"[2,4] which is based on the Global Northern conceptualization of SGD identity. Forcing SGD survival migrants to disclose their identity publicly may place them at risk for multilevel stigma, polyvictimization, and marginalization within their diaspora communities, creating a salient dissonance among those who have been intentional about survival by concealing their identity.[2,13,23] The social visibility dilemma is particularly pronounced given that it can occur when SGD survival

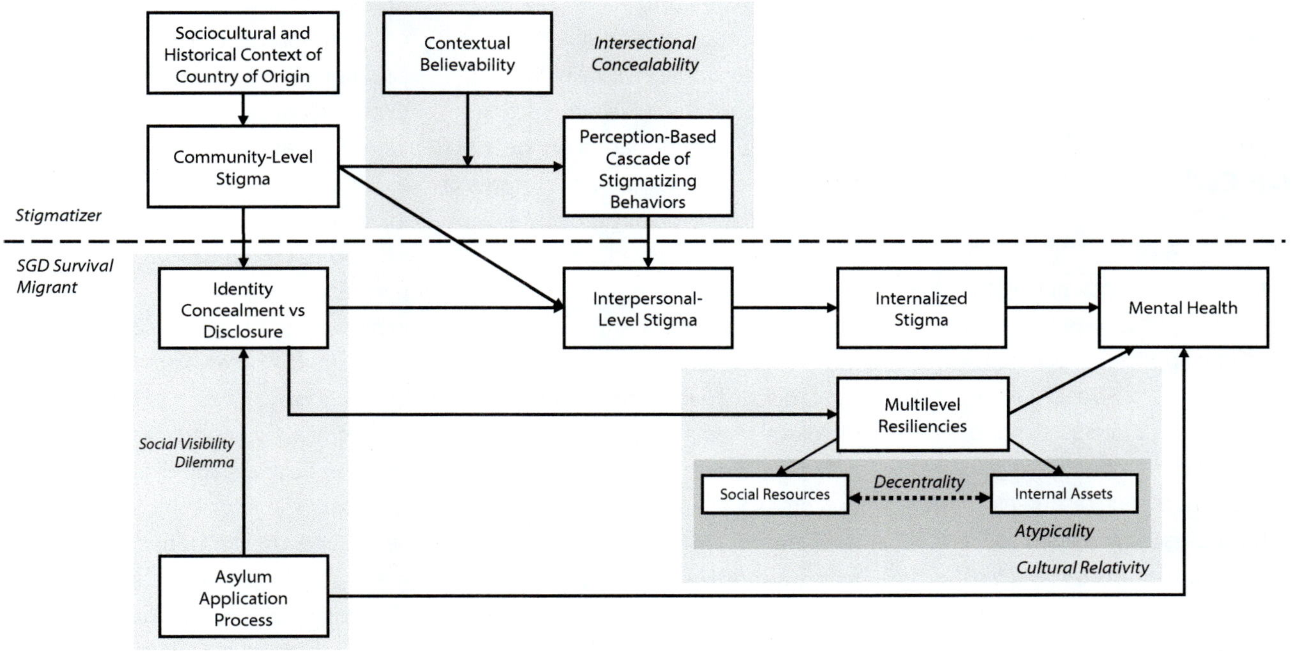

FIGURE 1— Atypical Resilience Conceptual Framework of Sexual and Gender-Diverse (SGD) Survival Migrants

migrants are in a socioeconomically precarious position.[2,4]

Aligned with the decentrality principle, which emphasizes the centrality of accessibility and availability of multilevel assets, the visibility dilemma undermines core interpersonal assets.[2,22] SGD survival migrants fleeing SGD-related prosecution are expected to openly integrate their SGD status to secure asylum protection in the United States, mostly without culturally congruent psychological support.[2,4] This disclosure for asylum petition must occur within 1 year of entering the country, which may pull identity expression out of its natural social and cultural context, imposing it on a timeline that may conflict with an individual's perceived readiness and safety.[2,11] Decentrality accentuates how stigma operates across multiple interacting domains.

To build a credible asylum case, SGD survival migrants must prove their SGD identity in ways that adjudicators deem credible while managing the risk of rejection, polyvictimization, or disconnection from their family or community networks.[2,22] They must also consider the repercussions for loved ones who remain in their country of origin, who could be victims of associated stigma.[13,15] Disclosure decisions must be timed and tailored to specific social contexts and audiences at the individual's autonomy rather than forcing an individual to consider social trade-offs.[4,23] Given current policies, inadequate visibility may lead to denied asylum, whereas premature or non-strategic disclosure can compromise safety, erode social support, trigger retraumatization, and provoke further polyvictimization.[2,13]

The atypicality principle is particularly relevant as SGD asylum seekers develop adaptive strategies that may appear as unconventional or counterintuitive approaches to overcoming an adverse circumstance.[21,22] Selective self-disclosure, strategic alignment with Global Northern SGD identity scripts, and cultural code switching are not signs of inauthenticity but rather sophisticated techniques for navigating conflicting demands.[4,23] These behaviors reflect resilience in the face of systemic pressures and structural stigma to conform to unfamiliar expectations around identity coherence.[6,11]

Cultural relativity brings attention to the disconnect between Global Northern assumptions about SGD identity and the diverse cultural contexts from which asylum seekers originate.[2,4] The US asylum system often expects consistent narratives and identity expressions modeled after Global Northern SGD frameworks.[4,13] However, these expectations may not match how SGD identities are understood, experienced, or expressed in other cultural settings.[4,23] As a result, applicants may be penalized for not exhibiting identity in ways adjudicators recognize as "authentic and credible," further compounding the visibility dilemma.[2,11]

INTERSECTIONAL CONCEALABILITY OF IDENTITY

Ultimately, the social visibility dilemma has enduring consequences beyond the asylum application process and across borders.[2,16] Decisions to be open about one's intersectional identities have implications for accessing multilevel resilience-supporting resources.[2,12] Identity disclosures may facilitate access to SGD-specific resources while also risking ostracism from diaspora communities or endangering family members in their country of origin.[4,13] Thus, strategic identity management becomes a chronic ecological adaptation rather than a one-time legal hurdle.[2,21,23] Viewing the social visibility dilemma through an ecological framework elucidates the structural constraints that shape SGD survival migrants' autonomy, agency, and resilience in social identity management.[21,22]

Another understudied stressor for this population is the concept of intersectional identity concealability.[6] Intersectional identity concealability is the idea that multiple stigmatized identities vary in how visible or concealable they are across migratory phases and contexts. This variability shapes individuals' exposure to stigma and their ability to access health-promoting resources and protections.[6,14,24] Unlike concealment, which refers to individuals' deliberate acts of withholding or disguising an identity, concealability describes how easily their social identities can be kept private or are likely to be perceived by others: put simply, the extent to which intersecting stigmatized identities are visible or identifiable to others, "passing as the norm."[6,23,24] Intersectional identity concealability differs from intersectional invisibility: when individuals with multiple intersecting minoritized identities are marginalized because they do not fit the prototypes of their constituent identity groups (e.g., able-presenting disabled individuals).[25]

In high-structural-stigma environments, intersecting identity concealability may help SGD survival migrants avoid discrimination, surveillance, and multilevel stigma cascades, including polyvictimization and other negative outcomes.[23,24] However, concealability is neither universally available nor uniformly protective, especially when identities intersect in ways that become more visible in specific contexts.[6,24] Concealability can prevent the first stigma cascade (labeling, acknowledgment, and awareness of multilevel intersectional stigma among SGD survival migrants).

Framing intersectional identity concealability through Ungar's social-ecological resilience theory provides a powerful lens for understanding how SGD survival migrants adapt to adversity.[11,22] Intersectional concealability of identity centers the source of harm: the multilevel stigma and social norms that create the permission structure and labeling of perceptions of intersecting stigmatized identities to constrain social determinants of health. It decenters the individual, which is what concealment does.[23,24] The principle of cultural relativity is especially relevant to understanding a central mechanism of intersectional concealability.

We propose 2 mechanisms of intersectional identity concealability: contextual believability and perception-based cascades. Contextual believability refers to the degree to which others accept a person's expressed or claimed identity as credible, authentic, or legitimate and how that acceptance varies across the migratory phases and social, cultural, or institutional settings.[6,14] It captures situations in which the same identity expression (e.g., coming out as gay, identifying as transgender, presenting as undocumented) might be validated in one context but doubted or rejected in another on the basis of the expectations and cultural frameworks of those in power. For instance, a gay man who maintained a heterosexual relationship in his country of origin to avoid multilevel stigma may have his asylum claim rejected because adjudicators perceive his sexual identity as uncredible. At the same time, the diaspora community might see the same case as credible or uncredible depending on the degree of concealability of SGD identity.

A second key mechanism is perception-based cascades, which refer to the chain of stigma-related consequences set into motion simply by how others perceive or categorize a person. These perceptions may be accurate or inaccurate, produced according to stereotypes; once activated, however, they can initiate a cascade of stigmatization and marginalizing responses (e.g., discrimination, social exclusion, denial of services, or targeted violence) that profoundly shape SGD survival migrants' access to rights, support, and safety. For example, a transgender woman may be perceived and labeled as transgender by a service provider on the basis of appearance or voice, triggering transnegative mistreatment even without verbal disclosure.[6,24] Similarly, an SGD survival migrant seeking asylum may be labeled as undocumented on the basis of accent, language use, or racial profiling, regardless of legal status. These perceptions, grounded in xenophobia and racism, are often outside the individual's control and shaped by societal biases. Yet, they profoundly shape SGD survival migrants' access to rights, resources, and safety by the propensity to unleash stigma cascades.[6,14,24]

PUBLIC HEALTH IMPLICATIONS

Taken together, these mechanisms illustrate how intersectional concealability is not simply a personal or behavioral issue but a structurally embedded condition that shapes both vulnerability and resilience. Leveraging Ungar's social-ecological resilience lens, we posit that the ability of SGD survival migrants to achieve optimal health outcomes and thrive depends not just on their own choices but on the availability, accessibility, and responsiveness of the multilevel assets around them.[11,22,24] Legal, health, and social service institutions must recognize that cultural norms, institutional expectations, and the affordances or constraints across the migratory phases shape identity navigation. What appears to be inconsistency or deception is often an expression of adaptation and resilience, an effort to survive within complex and often contradictory social environments.[11,22,24] SGD survival migrants' resilience must be seen for what it is: scar tissue emanating from high-structural-stigma environments and traumatogenic processes.[18,19]

CONCLUSIONS

This analytic essay provides arguments for understanding how SGD survival migrants leverage individual strengths and multilevel assets to progress from immediate survival to long-term flourishing. By examining these strategic navigations—especially social-visibility-dilemma and intersectional-identity-concealability processes—through an ecological lens, we shift the focus from viewing SGD survival migrants solely as victims to recognizing them as strategic actors navigating complex social ecologies in pursuit of environments that facilitate flourishing rather than merely survival. In addition, these intentional decisions are also often made to protect loved ones from associated stigma.

The current Immigration and Customs Enforcement raids and detentions typify intersectional identity concealability. The agency's arrests without due process are based on who its officials perceive as "documented" and "undocumented" irrespective of disclosed status. Understanding the strategic identity navigation processes of SGD survival migrants is essential for public health practitioners and policymakers seeking to develop effective, equity-driven responses. SGD survival migrants often face life-threatening risks when disclosing their sexual or gender identity and must carefully assess when, where, and to whom they can safely reveal this information. Equally, the intersectional concealability of their identity launches cascades of stigma or multilevel assets depending on the context. Public health efforts must prioritize culturally congruent mental health care, such as trauma-informed therapy offered by providers trained in both SGD and asylum medicine, and expand access to peer-led support networks grounded in the experiential expertise of SGD migrants.

At the policy level, current asylum processes often require detailed identity disclosure without adequate culturally congruent psychological support and privacy protections, placing applicants at greater risk for retraumatization, multilevel stigma, associated stigma for loved ones, and erosion of multilevel assets to support their flourishing after migration. Policy reforms should include removing the 1-year asylum petition limit, protecting asylum claim confidentiality, and validating identity beyond Global Northern SGD visibility norms. AJPH

ABOUT THE AUTHORS

David Chinyeaka Agor is with the Perelman School of Medicine Implementation Science Center and the School of Nursing, University of Pennsylvania, Philadelphia. Chioma Nnaji is with the Multicultural AIDS Coalition and Ocha Transformations, Boston, MA. Carmen Alvarez and Steven Meanley are with the School of Nursing, University of Pennsylvania. Jose Bauermeister is at the Perelman School of Medicine and the School of Nursing, University of Pennsylvania.

CORRESPONDENCE

Correspondence should be sent to David Chinyeaka Agor, DNP, 418 Curie Blvd 231L, Philadelphia, PA 19104 (e-mail: dagor@upenn.edu). Reprints can be ordered at https://www.ajph.org by clicking the "Reprints" link.

PUBLICATION INFORMATION

Full Citation: Agor DC, Nnaji C, Alvarez C, Bauermeister J, Meanley S. Unconventional resilience: necessary social identity management among asylum-seeking sexual and gender-diverse survival migrants. *Am J Public Health*. 2026;116(2):222–228.

Acceptance Date: October 18, 2025.

DOI: https://doi.org/10.2105/AJPH.2025.308337

ORCID IDs:

David Chinyeaka Agor https://orcid.org/0000-0002-3081-3585

Chioma Nnaji https://orcid.org/0000-0001-8512-7913

Jose Bauermeister https://orcid.org/0000-0002-9276-2306

Steven Meanley https://orcid.org/0000-0002-6098-9733

CONTRIBUTORS

The authors contributed equally to conception and design, analysis, drafting, and article revisions.

CONFLICTS OF INTEREST

The authors report no potential or actual conflicts of interest from funding or affiliation-related activities.

HUMAN PARTICIPANT PROTECTION

No protocol approval was required because this research did not involve human participants.

REFERENCES

1. Alessi EJ, Kahn S, Chatterji S. The darkest times of my life: recollections of child abuse among forced migrants persecuted because of their sexual orientation and gender identity. *Child Abuse Negl.* 2016;51:93–105. https://doi.org/10.1016/j.chiabu.2015.10.030
2. Piwowarczyk L, Fernandez P, Sharma A. Seeking asylum: challenges faced by the LGB community. *J Immigr Minor Health.* 2017;19(3):723–732. https://doi.org/10.1007/s10903-016-0363-9
3. Yarwood V, Checchi F, Lau K, Zimmerman C. LGBTQI + migrants: a systematic review and conceptual framework of health, safety and well-being during migration. *Int J Environ Res Public Health.* 2022;19(2):869. https://doi.org/10.3390/ijerph19020869
4. Fox SD, Griffin RH, Pachankis JE. Minority stress, social integration, and the mental health needs of LGBTQ asylum seekers in North America. *Soc Sci Med.* 2020;246:112727. https://doi.org/10.1016/j.socscimed.2019.112727
5. Flores AR. *Social Acceptance of LGBTI People in 175 Countries and Locations.* Los Angeles, CA: Williams Institute, UCLA School of Law; 2021.
6. Pachankis JE, Wang K. The conceptualizations, causes, and consequences of stigma: background for a model of migration-generated stigma. In: Yang LH, Eger MA, Link BG, eds. *Migration Stigma: Understanding Prejudice, Discrimination, and Exclusion.* Vol. 32. Cambridge, MA: MIT Press; 2024:69–73.
7. Hatzenbuehler ML. Structural stigma and health: how US policies mitigate and amplify stigma. In: Yang LH, Eger MA, Link BG, eds. *Migration Stigma: Understanding Prejudice, Discrimination, and Exclusion.* Vol. 32. Cambridge, MA: MIT Press; 2024: 166–171.
8. Pachankis JE, Hatzenbuehler ML, Berg RC, et al. Anti-LGBT and anti-immigrant structural stigma: an intersectional analysis of sexual minority men's HIV risk when migrating to or within Europe. *J Acquir Immune Defic Syndr.* 2017;76(4):356–366. https://doi.org/10.1097/QAI.0000000000001519
9. Agor D, Cargill V, Richie J. *Sexual and Gender-Diverse Survival Migration: A Blueprint for Action.* Washington, DC: Milken Institute, Public Health; 2024.
10. Betts A. Survival migration: A new protection framework. *Glob Governance.* 2010;16(3):361–382. Available at: https://www.jstor.org/stable/29764952. Accessed December 5, 2025.
11. Attia M, Das B, Tang S, Qiu Y, Li H, Nguyen C. Post-traumatic growth and resilience of LGBTQ+ asylum seekers in the United States. *Couns Psychol.* 2023;51(7):1005–1036. https://doi.org/10.1177/00110000231186112
12. Alessi EJ. Resilience in sexual and gender minority forced migrants: a qualitative exploration. *Traumatology.* 2016;22(3):203–213. https://doi.org/10.1037/trm0000077
13. Kahn S, Alessi EJ. Coming out under the gun: exploring the psychological dimensions of seeking refugee status for LGBT claimants in Canada. *J Refug Stud.* 2018;31(1):22–41. https://doi.org/10.1093/jrs/fex019
14. Blasco D, Link BG, Bohman A, et al. How are stigma processes related to different aspects of migration-generated diversity? In: Yang LH, Eger MA, Link BG, eds. *Migration Stigma: Understanding Prejudice, Discrimination, and Exclusion.* Vol. 32. Cambridge, MA: MIT Press; 2024:23–30.
15. Kahn S. Experiences of faith for gender role non-conforming Muslims in resettlement: preliminary considerations for social work practitioners. *Br J Soc Work.* 2015;45(7):2038–2055. Available at: https://www.jstor.org/stable/43687972. Accessed December 5, 2025.
16. Ibe-Lamberts K, Onyeise D. The effects of LGBTQ+ persecution on transnational African immigrants. *Am J Public Health.* 2025;115(8): 1236–1239. https://doi.org/10.2105/ajph.2025.308076
17. Teruya SA, Bazargan-Hejazi S. The immigrant and Hispanic paradoxes: a systematic review of their predictions and effects. *Hisp J Behav Sci.* 2013; 35(4):486–509. https://doi.org/10.1177/0739986313499004
18. Suslovic B, Lett E. Resilience is an adverse event: a critical discussion of resilience theory in health services research and public health. *Community Health Equity Res Policy.* 2024;44(3):339–343. https://doi.org/10.1177/2752535x231159721
19. Mahdiani H, Ungar M. The dark side of resilience. *Adv Res Sci.* 2021;2(3):147–155. https://doi.org/10.1007/s42844-021-00031-z
20. Rodríguez-Díaz CE. Community resistance as public health activism in Puerto Rico. *Am J Public Health.* 2020;110(10):1454–1455. https://doi.org/10.2105/AJPH.2020.305884
21. Ungar M. The social ecology of resilience: addressing contextual and cultural ambiguity of a nascent construct. *Am J Orthopsychiatry.* 2011;81(1):1–17. https://doi.org/10.1111/j.1939-0025.2010.01067.x
22. Ungar M. Resilience, trauma, context, and culture. *Trauma Violence Abuse.* 2013;14(3):255–266.
23. Pachankis JE, Mahon CP, Jackson SD, Fetzner BK, Bränström R. Sexual orientation concealment and mental health: a conceptual and meta-analytic review. *Psychol Bull.* 2020;146(10): 831–871. https://doi.org/10.1037/bul0000271
24. Quinn DM. When stigma is concealable: the costs and benefits for health. In: Major B, Dovidio JF, Link BG, eds. *The Oxford Handbook of Stigma, Discrimination, and Health.* New York, NY: Oxford University Press; 2018:287–297. https://doi.org/10.1093/oxfordhb/9780190243470.013.19
25. Coles SM, Pasek J. Intersectional invisibility revisited: how group prototypes lead to the erasure and exclusion of black women. *Transl Issues Psychol Sci.* 2020;6(4):314–324. https://psycnet.apa.org/doi/10.1037/tps0000256

Association Between Gender Affirmation and Adoption Interest Among a Large Sample of Transgender, Nonbinary, and Gender-Diverse Populations in Washington State, 2023

Adedotun Ogunbajo, PhD, MPH, Teresa DeAtley, PhD, MHS, Aaron Breslow, MPH, Kristi Gamarel, PhD, Don Operario, PhD, EdM, Trace Kershaw, PhD, Rebecca L. Emery Tavernier, PhD, and Arjee Javellana Restar, PhD, MPH

See also LGBTQ+ Well-Being and Joy, pp. 188–250.

Objectives. To investigate the association between gender affirmation and interest in adoption among transgender, nonbinary, and gender-diverse adults.

Methods. We analyzed data from the Washington Priority Assessment in Trans Health Project, which was conducted in Washington State in 2023. We controlled for sociodemographic characteristics and health care indicators using multinomial logistic regression.

Results. Of the 788 participants, 56% expressed interest in adoption, 24% were undecided or maybe interested, and 20% reported no interest. Participants who expressed interest in adoption were more likely to have updated their legal name documentation (adjusted odds ratio [AOR] = 4.7; 95% confidence interval [CI] = 2.73, 8.08), were more likely to have private insurance (AOR = 11.01; 95% CI = 2.89, 42.02), and were less likely to have food insecurity (AOR = 0.46; 95% CI = 0.20, 0.82). Participants who were undecided about adoption reported higher rates of legal gender affirmation (AOR = 1.59; 95% CI = 1.04, 2.42), educational attainment (AOR = 3.77; 95% CI = 1.19, 11.91), and internalized transphobia (AOR = 1.53; 95% CI = 1.01, 2.34).

Conclusions. Legal gender affirmation and health care access were associated with adoption interest and were significantly influenced by economic stability and psychological factors. Comprehensive initiatives are needed to develop more trans-inclusive family-planning services. (*Am J Public Health*. 2026;116(2):229–239. https://doi.org/10.2105/AJPH.2025.308312)

AJPH February 2026, Vol. 116, No. 2

Parenting desires and intentions and patterns of family formation are largely understudied among sexual and gender minority populations, with most previous research conducted among lesbian, gay, and bisexual individuals and limited research on transgender, nonbinary, and gender-diverse (trans) communities.[1,2] A systematic review on the parenting desires and intentions among trans communities found that 48% to 75% desired genetically related children, and 51% to 94% were interested in child adoption.[3–5] Factors that influence desires and intentions for parenting among trans people include age, being in a relationship, financial stability, a supportive relationship with family, and an existing biological child.[3]

Gender affirmation, encompassing psychological, social, medical, and legal dimensions, is crucial for the well-being of trans individuals and for supporting their family-formation decisions.[6–8] Psychological affirmation, including positive self-regard and reduced internalized transphobia, improved mental health outcomes and greater confidence in pursuing parenthood.[9] Social affirmation through familial support and community acceptance significantly influences trans individuals' ability to navigate major life transitions and access to resources,[10] including family-building resources.[11] Medical gender affirmation, including hormone therapy and surgeries, is associated with improved quality of life and increased engagement with health care systems that can support family planning.[6,12–14] Legal gender affirmation, such as an updated name and gender marker on government identification documents, can reduce discrimination and mistreatment[15] and aid in adoption or other family-formation services.[16] These forms of gender affirmation may be relevant to adoption interest, as they can affect the sense of preparedness for parenthood and perceived ability to navigate adoption systems successfully.

Research on inclusive family-building policies for trans individuals remains critically limited despite increasing recognition of diverse family structures.[11] Many trans individuals face substantial barriers, including inconsistent legal protections across states, varying agency policies regarding trans adoptive parents, and limited cultural competency among adoption professionals.[11,17,18] These gaps in services are particularly concerning, given the documented interest in adoption among trans communities and the societal benefits of supporting diverse family formations.[5] Understanding the correlates of adoption interest among transgender individuals is essential for informing the development of inclusive family-building policies and support services.

We investigated the association between various forms of gender affirmation—psychological, social, medical, and legal—along with socioeconomic factors, health care access, and adoption interest among a large sample of trans individuals in Washington State. We hypothesized that higher levels of gender affirmation would be associated with increased interest in adoption. We sought to contribute to a more comprehensive understanding of family-formation pathways in trans communities and to inform interventions that support trans individuals in achieving their family-building goals.

METHODS

We drew on data from the Washington Priority Assessment in Trans Health Project, a cross-sectional survey that was designed with, for, and by trans and nonbinary residents of Washington State between March and April 2023 ($n = 788$). The survey explored various health topics, and we focused on the survey domains related to adoption interest.

As discussed in more detail elsewhere,[19,20] recruitment employed community-based strategies through partnerships with local LGBTQ+ (lesbian, gay, bisexual, transgender, queer, questioning, asexual, intersex, and other nonheterosexual, noncisgender) organizations, trans-led community groups, and health care providers serving transgender and nonbinary populations. Outreach was conducted through advisory board networks composed of transgender community members and advocates, community listservs, support groups, and social media platforms. The advisory board guided recruitment strategies to reach diverse segments of the trans community across Washington State.

Participants were eligible if they (1) were aged 18 years or older, (2) identified as transgender or nonbinary, (3) currently resided in Washington State, and (4) provided electronic consent. The survey adhered to best research practices for online surveys. The survey incorporated measures to minimize participant burden, such as limiting the completion time to 25 to 30 minutes and enabling an automatic save feature.

Measures

To assess adoption interest, we asked participants: "Are you interested in adopting a child?" with the response options "yes," "no," or "undecided/maybe." Given the lack of validated measures to assess gender affirmation, the development of the survey proceeded by cocreating questions with the study's advisory board members, who were deemed able to determine these dimensions directly.[21]

To assess internalized transphobia and trans acceptance, we asked participants whether they (1) were glad that they were trans, and (2) felt accepted by other trans people. Responses were treated continuously via a 5-point Likert scale with 1 = strongly disagree to 5 = strongly agree. We assessed family support and the proportion of families that supported participants' gender identity as dimensions of social affirmation. To evaluate the level of family support we asked, "How supportive of your gender identity/expression is your family?" with response options treated dichotomously as 0 = not very/not at all supportive and 1 = very/somewhat supportive. To assess the proportion of supportive family members, we asked, "Thinking about your entire family members, what proportion of your family is supportive of your gender identity/expression?" with response categories of 0 = less than a half, 1 = about

AJPH February 2026, Vol. 116, No. 2

half, and 2 = more than a half or all of them.

We assessed the history of medical gender-affirming care and current hormone therapy use for transition (yes/no) or any history of gender-affirming care surgery (yes/no). We limited the responses to those whose gender goals included these medical gender-affirming care services. We assessed participants' history of legal gender affirmation by asking which major government identification documents they had updated: (1) name, and (2) gender marker. We limited responses to those whose gender goals included these legal gender affirmation options.

Covariates included sociodemographic data (i.e., age, gender identity, race/ethnicity, sexual orientation, educational attainment, residential geography, living below or above the state-defined poverty level, and current employment status). Responses are summarized in Table 1. We assessed additional variables related to health care, housing, and food security. Health care indicators included types of insurance (public, private, or not sure/do not know), history of past year routine examination (yes/no), and any previous discussion of fertility options with a health care provider (yes/no). We derived food insecurity questions from the US Household Food Security Survey Module,[22] which included 4 questions asking participants to indicate whether they had enough food, they were worried that their food would run out, they were worried that the food they bought would not last, or they were worried that they would run out of money to buy more food when needed in the past 12 months. We summed responses based on the Likert scale option of 1 = often true, 2 = sometimes true, and 3 = never true. Lastly, we asked about the participants' living status and whether they were a current homeowner, were a renter or lessee, or were living in another housing situation.

Data Analysis

We conducted descriptive analyses to summarize the distribution of variables and bivariate analyses to explore independent relationships among the independent variables, covariates, and adoption interest. We used the χ^2 test for categorical independent variables and analysis of variance for continuous independent variables to assess the significance of these relationships at the bivariate level. To delineate characteristics associated with adoption interest, we conducted multivariable multinomial logistic regression analyses with "not interested in adoption" as the reference category, including all independent variables and covariates in the model.

We ran a variance inflation factor analysis to detect multicollinearity[23] and removed the following variables to reduce collinearity: assigned sex at birth, sexual orientation, and legal gender. To address potential model instability from the modest sample size, we applied nonparametric bootstrapping with 1000 iterations to estimate confidence intervals (CIs) for the final adjusted model. We examined missing data patterns and found that they were minimal (< 5%). We employed a comprehensive case analysis to develop models.

The final model included 756 participants with complete data and achieved a pseudo R^2 of 0.28, indicating adequate model performance. We set statistical significance at an α level of less than 0.05 a priori. We performed all analyses using Stata MP version 17.0 (StataCorp LP, College Station, TX).

RESULTS

Participants' sociodemographic characteristics are provided in Table 1 (n = 788); 56% expressed interest in adoption, 24% were undecided or maybe interested, and 20% were not interested.

Participant Characteristics

Participants who expressed interest in adoption were significantly older, with a mean age of 30 years, compared with 27 years in the other groups (P < .001). There were notable differences in gender identity by interest in adoption. Among respondents who expressed interest in adoption, 82.2% were transgender women. Among transgender women, 65.6% expressed interest in adoption, compared with 14.7% among transgender men and 6.2% among nonbinary individuals. Similarly, individuals assigned male at birth overwhelmingly expressed being interested in adoption (97%) compared with those assigned female at birth (3.2%). Among individuals assigned male at birth, 64.6% were interested in adoption, whereas 44.2% of individuals assigned female at birth were interested in adoption. Heterosexual participants (44%) and gay, lesbian, same gender–attracted participants (53%) were more likely to express interest in adoption than were bisexual (2%) and queer (1%) individuals.

A higher percentage of non-Hispanic White participants (58%) reported interest in adoption compared with non-Hispanic Asian/Asian American (15%), non-Hispanic Black/African American (15%), and Hispanic/Latine (12%) participants. Adoption interest varied by residential geography, with individuals living in a large city reporting more interest in adoption (26%) compared with

AJPH February 2026, Vol. 116, No. 2

TABLE 1— Sociodemographic Characteristics and Gender Affirmation Factors by Adoption Interest Among Transgender, Nonbinary, and Gender-Diverse Adults: Washington Priority Assessment in Trans Health Project, Washington State, 2023

	Overall, No. (%) or Mean ±SD	Is Not Interested, No. (%) or Mean ±SD	Is Interested, No. (%) or Mean ±SD	Might Be Interested, No. (%) or Mean ±SD	P
Total sample	788 (100)	161 (20.4)	440 (55.8)	187 (23.7)	
Sociodemographic characteristics					
Age, y	28.9 ±4.4	27.1 ±6.2	30.3 ±3.1	27.2 ±4.0	≤.001
Gender identity					<.001
Woman, including transgender woman	648 (82.2)	96 (59.6)	425 (96.6)	127 (67.9)	
Man, including transgender man	75 (9.5)	32 (19.9)	11 (2.5)	32 (17.1)	
Nonbinary, including gender nonconforming, Two-Spirit	65 (8.3)	33 (19.3)	4 (0.9)	28 (15.0)	
Sex assigned at birth					<.001
Assigned male at birth	659 (83.6)	105 (63.4)	426 (96.8)	131 (70.0)	
Assigned female at birth	122 (15.5)	54 (33.5)	14 (3.2)	54 (28.9)	
Intersex	7 (0.9)	5 (3.1)	. . .	2 (1.1)	
Sexual orientation					<.001
Straight/heterosexual	303 (38.5)	16 (9.9)	193 (43.8)	94 (50.3)	
Gay/lesbian/same-gender attracted	339 (43.0)	75 (46.6)	233 (53.0)	31 (16.6)	
Bisexual	64 (8.0)	32 (19.9)	9 (2.0)	23 (12.3)	
Queer	65 (8.3)	30 (18.6)	3 (0.7)	32 (17.1)	
Another sexual orientation	17 (2.2)	8 (4.9)	2 (0.5)	7 (3.7)	
Race/ethnicity					.09
Non-Hispanic White	474 (60.2)	96 (60.0)	253 (57.5)	125 (66.8)	
Person of color	313 (39.8)	64 (40.0)	187 (42.5)	62 (33.2)	
Non-Hispanic Asian/Asian American	88 (11.2)	14 (8.6)	65 (14.8)	9 (4.8)	<.001
Non-Hispanic Black/African American	102 (12.9)	18 (11.3)	65 (14.8)	19 (10.2)	
Hispanic/Latine/Spanish origin	69 (8.8)	8 (5.0)	53 (12.0)	8 (4.2)	
Non-Hispanic Middle Eastern/North African	7 (0.9)	4 (2.5)	1 (0.2)	2 (1.1)	
Non-Hispanic Native Hawaiian/Pacific Islander	10 (1.3)	7 (4.4)	1 (0.2)	2 (1.1)	
Non-Hispanic American Indian/Alaska Native	10 (1.3)	4 (2.5)	. . .	6 (3.2)	
Multiple race/ethnicity	27 (3.4)	9 (5.6)	2 (0.5)	16 (8.6)	
Residential geography					<.001
Large city	303 (38.5)	108 (67.1)	116 (26.4)	79 (42.2)	
Rural area	103 (13.1)	1 (0.6)	100 (22.7)	2 (1.1)	
Small city/town	226 (28.7)	37 (23.0)	101 (23.0)	88 (47.1)	
Suburb near large city	156 (19.8)	15 (9.3)	123 (28.0)	18 (9.6)	
Education attained					<.001
≤high school	422 (53.6)	60 (37.3)	365 (60.2)	97 (51.8)	
Some college/technical school	276 (35.0)	65 (40.4)	161 (36.6)	50 (26.7)	
College/graduate school	90 (11.4)	36 (22.3)	14 (3.2)	40 (21.4)	
Living below poverty level					<.001
No	641 (81.4)	102 (63.4)	433 (98.4)	106 (56.7)	
Yes	147 (18.6)	59 (36.6)	7 (1.6)	81 (43.3)	

Continued

TABLE 1— Continued

	Overall, No. (%) or Mean ±SD	Is Not Interested, No. (%) or Mean ±SD	Is Interested, No. (%) or Mean ±SD	Might Be Interested, No. (%) or Mean ±SD	P
Current employment status					<.001
Not employed	21 (2.7)	10 (6.2)	4 (0.9)	7 (3.7)	
Employed	767 (97.3)	151 (93.8)	436 (99.1)	180 (96.3)	
Psychological affirmation					
Internalized transphobia (min = 1; max = 5)	1.9 ±0.9	2.19 ±1.0	1.6 ±0.7	2.4 ±0.9	≤.001
Felt accepted by other trans members (min = 1; max = 5)	3.9 ±0.8	3.8 ±0.8	4.0 ±0.8	3.6 ±0.8	≤.001
Social affirmation					
Level of family support					<.001
Not very/not at all supportive	236 (30.1)	54 (34.0)	156 (35.5)	26 (13.9)	
Very/somewhat supportive	550 (69.9)	105 (66.0)	284 (64.5)	161 (86.1)	
Proportion of supportive family					<.001
<half	197 (25.1)	40 (25.2)	138 (31.4)	19 (10.2)	
~half	283 (36.0)	55 (34.6)	158 (35.9)	70 (37.4)	
>half/all	306 (38.9)	64 (40.2)	144 (32.7)	98 (52.4)	
Medical affirmation					
Currently receiving hormone therapy if wanted (n = 636)					<.001
No	134 (21.1)	68 (65.4)	12 (2.7)	54 (58.1)	
Yes	502 (78.9)	36 (34.6)	427 (97.3)	39 (41.9)	
Received gender-affirming surgery if wanted (n = 609)					<.001
No	88 (14.6)	45 (52.9)	8 (1.8)	35 (42.7)	
Yes	514 (85.4)	40 (47.1)	427 (98.2)	47 (57.3)	
Legal affirmation					
Updated gender on ID documents if wanted (n = 770; min = 0; max = 4)	2.7 ±1.7	0.9 ±1.1	3.9 ±0.7	1.2 ±1.3	≤.001
Updated name on ID documents if wanted (n = 751; min = 0; max = 4)	2.8 ±1.6	1.0 ±1.2	3.9 ±0.6	1.4 ±1.3	≤.001
Awareness of trans policy environment					
Awareness of antitransgender bills in the US (min = 1; max = 5)	3.15 ±1.09	2.9 ±1.1	3.4 ±1.1	2.9 ±1.0	<.001
Worried about rights being taken away					<.001
Yes	365 (46.3)	86 (53.4)	220 (50.0)	59 (31.6)	
No	423 (53.7)	75 (46.6)	220 (50.0)	128 (68.5)	
Health care access					
Health insurance type					<.001
Public insurance (Medicare, Medicaid)	163 (20.7)	93 (57.8)	17 (3.9)	53 (28.3)	
Private insurance	622 (78.9)	66 (41.0)	423 (96.1)	133 (71.2)	
Don't know/not sure	3 (0.4)	2 (1.2)	...	1 (0.5)	
Past year routine examination					<.001
No	66 (8.4)	28 (17.7)	6 (1.4)	32 (17.3)	
Yes	717 (91.6)	130 (82.3)	434 (98.6)	153 (82.7)	
Discussed fertility options with provider					<.001
No, and do not want to	373 (49.7)	130 (9.3)	211 (48.2)	32 (19.0)	
No, but would like to	322 (42.9)	1 (0.7)	215 (49.1)	106 (62.7)	
Yes	56 (7.4)	13 (9.0)	12 (2.7)	31 (18.3)	

Continued

TABLE 1— Continued

	Overall, No. (%) or Mean ±SD	Is Not Interested, No. (%) or Mean ±SD	Is Interested, No. (%) or Mean ±SD	Might Be Interested, No. (%) or Mean ±SD	P
Household and food security					
Food insecurity (min = 0; max = 3)	0.4 ±0.9	0.8 ±1.2	0.1 ±0.4	0.6 ±1.1	<.001
Living status					<.001
Homeowner	260 (33.0)	23 (14.3)	215 (48.9)	22 (11.8)	
Renter/lessee	450 (57.1)	98 (60.9)	221 (50.2)	131 (70.0)	
Other housing	78 (9.9)	40 (24.8)	4 (0.9)	34 (18.2)	

Note: We used analysis of variance to test mean age differences and the χ^2 test to test difference in categorical outcomes between 3 groups.

individuals residing in a small city or town (23%) or rural area (23%). The majority (60%) of those with elementary to high school education attainment were interested in adoption, whereas only 37% and 3% of participants with some college or graduate school education, respectively, expressed interest. Among those interested in adoption, 98% were above the poverty line, and 99% reported being employed.

Internalized transphobia scores were higher among those not interested in or undecided about adoption, with individuals reporting interest in adoption having lower internalized transphobia scores ($P<.001$). Supportive family environments were also more common among the interested group, with 65% reporting having very or somewhat supportive families ($P<.001$).

Medical and legal affirmation variables were associated with adoption interest. Participants interested in adoption were significantly more likely to have received gender-affirming care, including hormone therapy and surgeries (97% and 98%, respectively) compared with those who were not interested in adoption (35% and 47%, respectively). Legal affirmation (e.g., updating gender and name on identification documents) was also more common among those interested in adoption than those not interested or undecided about adoption ($P<.001$).

Having private insurance coverage was more common among those interested in adoption (96%), whereas having public insurance was more frequent among those not interested in or undecided about adoption. The vast majority (99%) of those interested in adoption reported having had a routine health care examination in the past year, compared with 82% and 83% of those in the not interested and undecided groups, respectively. Food insecurity was most prevalent among those not interested in or undecided about adoption compared with those in the interested group ($P<.001$). Participants who were interested in adoption reported higher rates of homeownership (49%) and lower rates of renting or living in other housing situations.

Multivariable Analyses

Compared with those not interested in adoption, participants interested in adoption had 5 times the odds of having their name updated on their legal identification documents (adjusted odds ratio (AOR) = 4.7; 95% CI = 2.73, 8.08), 11 times the odds of having private insurance vs public insurance (AOR = 11.01; 95% CI = 2.89, 42.02), and nearly 20 times the odds of having discussed fertility options with providers versus not (AOR = 19.2; 95% CI = 2.38, 154.51). Compared with those not interested in adoption, participants interested in adoption had lower odds of having experienced food insecurity (AOR = 0.46; 95% CI = 0.20, 0.82). Lastly, interested participants had lower odds of having lived in other housing situations versus being homeowners (AOR = 0.06; 95% CI = 0.01, 0.67) compared with those not interested in adoption.

Similarly, participants who were undecided about adoption had higher odds than did those who were not interested in adoption of having their name updated on their legal identification documents (AOR = 1.59; 95% CI = 1.04, 2.42). Additionally, compared with those not interested in adoption, undecided participants had higher odds of having attained some college or technical school education versus elementary or high school (AOR = 3.77; 95% CI = 1.19, 11.91) and were more likely to display higher internalized transphobia (AOR = 1.53; 95% CI = 1.01, 2.34). However, this association was modest compared with other factors in the model.

TABLE 2— **Multivariable Multinomial Logistic Regression of Adoption Interest Among Transgender, Nonbinary, and Gender-Diverse Adults: Washington Priority Assessment in Trans Health Project, Washington State, 2023**

Total Sample	Is Interested (Compared With Not Interested), AOR (95% CI) or Mean ±SD	Might Be Interested (Compared With Not Interested), AOR (95% CI) or Mean ±SD
Sociodemographic characteristics		
Age, y	0.91 ±0.82	0.92 ±0.85
Gender identity		
Woman, including transgender woman (Ref)	1	1
Man, including transgender man	2.53 (0.47, 13.55)	1.93 (0.61, 6.05)
Nonbinary, including gender nonconforming, Two-Spirit	0.54 (0.05, 5.42)	1.67 (0.48, 5.74)
Race/ethnicity		
Non-Hispanic White (Ref)	1	1
Person of color	1.53 (0.48, 4.81)	1.05 (0.42, 2.64)
Residential geography		
Large city (Ref)	1	1
Rural area	2.80 (0.18, 41.83)	1.03 (0.05, 20.51)
Small city/town	0.43 (0.12, 1.60)	1.02 (0.34, 2.03)
Suburb near large city	1.92 (0.44, 8.32)	1.08 (0.34, 3.48)
Education attained		
≤high school (Ref)	1	1
Some college/technical school	2.04 (0.52, 7.95)	3.77 (1.19, 11.91)
College/graduate school	0.35 (0.06, 2.07)	2.83 (0.72, 11.00)
Living below poverty level		
No (Ref)	1	1
Yes	0.50 (0.09, 2.64)	2.39 (0.83, 6.81)
Current employment status		
Not employed (Ref)	1	1
Employed	0.11 (0.01, 1.21)	0.60 (0.10, 3.41)
Psychological affirmation		
Internalized transphobia	1.15 (0.62, 2.13)	1.53 (1.01, 2.34)
Felt accepted by others	1.22 (0.65, 2.27)	1.40 (0.84, 2.34)
Social affirmation		
Level of family support		
Not very/not at all supportive (Ref)	1	1
Very/somewhat supportive	0.66 (0.19, 2.25)	0.59 (0.21, 1.67)
Proportion of supportive family		
< half (Ref)	1	1
~half	1.48 (0.35, 6.26)	2.46 (0.74, 8.06)
> half/all	0.96 (0.24, 3.74)	2.50 (0.73, 8.52)
Medical affirmation		
Currently receiving hormone therapy if wanted		
No (Ref)	1	1
Yes	2.06 (0.42, 10.03)	0.95 (0.29, 3.14)
Received gender-affirming surgery if wanted		
No (Ref)	1	1
Yes	0.68 (0.12, 3.73)	1.34 (0.41, 4.37)

Continued

TABLE 2— Continued

Total Sample	Is Interested (Compared With Not Interested), AOR (95% CI) or Mean ±SD	Might Be Interested (Compared With Not Interested), AOR (95% CI) or Mean ±SD
	Legal affirmation	
Updated name on ID documents if wanted	4.7 (2.73, 8.08)	1.59 (1.04, 2.42)
	Awareness of trans policy environment	
Awareness of antitransgender bills in the United States	1.07 (0.63, 1.83)	0.85 (0.54, 1.34)
Worried about rights being taken away		
No (Ref)	1	1
Yes	0.56 (0.18, 1.71)	1.39 (0.55, 3.52)
	Health care access	
Health insurance type		
Public insurance (Medicare, Medicaid) (Ref)	1	1
Private insurance	11.01 (2.89, 42.02)	1.10 (0.41, 2.97)
Past year routine examination		
No (Ref)	1	1
Yes	1.71 (0.32, 8.91)	1.21 (0.43, 3.38)
Discussed fertility options with provider		
No (Ref)	1	1
Yes	19.2 (2.38, 154.51)	2.97 (0.80, 10.98)
	Household and food security	
Food insecurity	0.46 (0.20, 0.82)	0.72 (0.44,1.18)
Living status		
Homeowner (Ref)	1	1
Renter/lessee	0.76 (0.21, 2.69)	0.56 (0.16, 1.90)
Other housing	0.06 (0.01, 0.67)	0.77 (0.20, 2.96)

Note. AOR = adjusted odds ratio; CI = confidence interval. We removed assigned sex at birth, sexual orientation, and legal gender from the model after testing for multicollinearity via variance inflation factor procedures. We ran the model with bootstrapping procedures of 1000 iterations.

AJPH February 2026, Vol. 116, No. 2

DISCUSSION

This study is among the first comprehensive investigations of the association among various dimensions of gender affirmation and interest in adoption among trans people. Our findings reveal significant associations between adoption interest and multiple forms of gender affirmation, particularly legal recognition, gender-affirming resources, and support systems, including health care access. Our results highlight how systemic factors can shape family-formation pathways and opportunities for trans communities. These results are particularly significant given the current political and social landscape constraining both trans rights and adoption access,[18] suggesting that any effort to support trans individuals in family formation must address multiple interconnected barriers.

Our findings reveal that legal gender affirmation was strongly correlated with adoption interest among trans persons. This likely reflects both practical and psychological dimensions of the adoption process. Legal gender affirmation may provide individuals with a sense of legitimacy and preparedness to navigate the complex legal requirements of adoption, while potentially reducing barriers[15] to discrimination when engaging with adoption agency policies and state-level family laws.[18] Future research on how gender markers and name change policies could facilitate adoption might provide insights into improving inclusivity and support for trans individuals seeking to adopt.

We found that health care resource access and provider support play crucial roles in shaping interest in adoption. This suggests that broader access to comprehensive health care may facilitate the exploration of family-building options.[24] These findings align with previous research highlighting the importance of provider–patient relationships and health care access in supporting family planning among sexual and gender minority individuals.[11,12,16,18] The higher likelihood of adoption interest among those who have discussed fertility options with providers underscores the critical role of health care providers in facilitating discussions about family formation. Given this finding, there is a need to cultivate provider training in discussing fertility options and adoption comprehensively with trans patients,[25–28] which could facilitate trans people's informed decisions about their family-building journey, ensuring that all options are explored and supported.

Socioeconomic stability also emerged as a key factor influencing adoption interest, as evidenced by the relationships between adoption interest and proxy variables of stable socioeconomic status, including higher educational attainment, food security, homeownership, and private insurance. These associations likely reflect both the practical and financial requirements of adoption processes—which often involve significant costs and home evaluations—and the broader impact of economic security on family-planning decisions.[29] The finding that participants experiencing fewer economic hardships are more interested in adoption highlights the need for policies addressing economic instabilities and financial barriers to adoption for trans individuals.[11] The link between socioeconomic stability and adoption interest also highlights the importance of financially inclusive, family-centered programs and policies in effectively addressing economic barriers to family planning. Ensuring eligibility for paid parental leave among trans employees who are new parents is crucial.[30,31] Clear policy guidelines and broader awareness of such provisions can significantly reduce financial and economic strains related to employment security and support trans people's family-formation goals.

Our findings also reveal substantial differences in adoption interest by gender identity that warrant specific attention. The stark contrast between transgender women (65.6% expressing interest) and transgender men (14.7% expressing interest) may reflect how reproductive anatomy influences family-formation preferences. Transgender men may have pregnancy options and access to biological parenthood that transgender women do not, potentially affecting their consideration of adoption as a primary family-formation pathway. This difference, although consistent with sex assigned at birth patterns, highlights the need for family-building counseling approaches that acknowledge these distinct reproductive realities and options. Future research should explore how different gender identities approach family-formation decisions and what specific support services might be most beneficial for each gender group.

Lastly, the association between potential adoption interest and higher internalized transphobia reveals complex psychological dynamics that trans individuals navigate when considering parenthood.[9,26,32] This relationship may reflect how internalized stigma creates ambivalence about parenting roles, as individuals grapple with societal messages about who can or should be parents.[5,32] Research suggests that trans individuals often face unique psychological challenges when contemplating parenthood, including concerns about their ability to provide stable parenting, fears of discrimination affecting their children, and anxiety about how their gender identity might affect their children's social experiences.[5,33]

The modest association with internalized transphobia among those expressing uncertainty, rather than definitive interest or disinterest, may indicate a state of contemplation in which individuals are actively processing these complex emotions and societal messages. This finding underscores the critical need for adoption services to incorporate trans-competent mental health support that specifically addresses internalized transphobia, parenting anxieties, and family-building concerns.[34] Furthermore, it suggests that psychological support services should be available not only during the adoption process but also during the early stages of family planning when individuals are first considering their parenting options.[34]

It should be emphasized that comprehensive pre-adoption counseling and support services would benefit all prospective adopting parents, including those already expressing interest in adoption, given the complex considerations involved in any adoption process. Lastly, more upstream approaches such as comprehensive sex education aiming to normalize different family dynamics and public health campaigns that prominently feature trans parents with the goal of reducing stigma are needed.

Limitations

This study has several limitations. Although the cross-sectional design prevents causal inference about the relationships between gender affirmation and adoption interest, the associations identified are valuable for informing policy and practice development. The sample, although diverse across sociodemographic factors, was a convenience sample from Washington State, a relatively liberal state with supportive LGBTQ+ policies, and may not represent trans individuals in more conservative states.

A significant limitation was our inability to account for existing children (biological or adopted), which could substantially influence adoption interest and is an important factor in interpreting these findings. Additionally, our measure of adoption interest captures current intentions but may not reflect future behavior or account for the dynamic nature of family-building decisions. Also, the measure is only 1 indicator of adoption interest, and we did not assess other aspects of family planning. Rather than treating the single-item adoption measure solely as a limitation to be remedied in future studies, our focus on adoption interest offers meaningful insight. For many trans individuals, adoption remains the most accessible and realistic path to family formation, given the substantial financial and logistical barriers to other assisted reproductive technologies. Additionally, our analysis was limited by not capturing important contextual factors that could influence adoption interest, such as current relationship status, partner gender identity and preferences, and existing children in the household.

Our focus on individual-level characteristics may not fully capture systemic barriers in adoption systems or variations in state-level policies that affect trans individuals' adoption experiences. Future research comparing state-level policies and their effects on family formation would provide valuable insights for policy development. Furthermore, our measures of gender affirmation, although comprehensive, might not have captured all relevant aspects of affirmation[8,35] or the nuanced ways these experiences interact with adoption interest.

Our reliance on self-reported data might also have introduced social desirability bias, particularly for sensitive topics such as family planning and gender identity. The wide CIs observed in some analyses reflect the complexity of the models and modest sample sizes for certain subgroups. Retaining all theoretically important variables in the final model enabled a more complete examination of gender affirmation dimensions; however, this approach may also have introduced additional model complexity and resulted in wider CIs. Future research with larger sample sizes might benefit from more parsimonious modeling approaches. Longitudinal research examining how gender affirmation relates to actual adoption outcomes would also provide valuable insights, as would studies incorporating partner perspectives, institutional policies, and geographic variations in adoption access.

Conclusions

This study demonstrates that adoption interest among trans individuals is strongly associated with multiple dimensions of gender affirmation, particularly legal recognition and health care access, and is significantly influenced by economic stability and psychological factors. Our findings have several important public health implications.

First, health care systems should prioritize comprehensive training for providers in discussing family-formation options, including adoption, with trans patients. Second, public health initiatives should focus on reducing economic barriers to adoption through targeted economic or financial assistance programs that explicitly include trans parents in existing family support systems, given the clear relationship between economic stability and adoption interest. Third, mental health services specifically addressing internalized transphobia and parenting concerns should be integrated into adoption services and made available during the early stages of family planning. As states continue to shape policies affecting both trans rights and adoption access, these findings underscore the need for coordinated efforts across health care, legal, and social service sectors to create more inclusive and supportive pathways to family formation for trans individuals. Future research and policy development should prioritize addressing these interconnected barriers and work to ensure that family-building support systems explicitly include and are accessible to trans communities. AJPH

ABOUT THE AUTHORS

Adedotun Ogunbajo is with the RAND Corporation, Santa Monica, CA. Teresa DeAtley is with the University of Utah School of Medicine, Salt Lake City. Aaron Breslow was with the Department of Psychiatry and Behavioral Sciences, Albert Einstein College of Medicine, Bronx, NY, at the time of the study. Kristi Gamarel is with the Department of Health Behavior and Health Equity, University of Michigan School of Public Health, Ann Arbor. Don Operario is with the Department of Behavioral, Social, and Health Education Sciences, Emory University Rollins School of Public Health, Atlanta, GA. Trace Kershaw is with the Department of Social and Behavioral Sciences, Yale University School of Public Health, New Haven, CT. Rebecca L. Emery Tavernier is with the Weitzman Institute, Moses/Weitzman Healthcare System, Middletown, CT. Arjee Javellana Restar was with the Departments of Epidemiology and Health Systems and Population Health, University of Washington School of Public Health, Seattle, at the time of the study.

CORRESPONDENCE

Correspondence should be sent to Adedotun Ogunbajo, 1200 S Hayes St, Arlington, VA 22202 (e-mail: dotunogunbajo@gmail.com). Reprints can be ordered at https://www.ajph.org by clicking the "Reprints" link.

PUBLICATION INFORMATION

Full Citation: Ogunbajo A, DeAtley T, Breslow A, et al. Association between gender affirmation and adoption interest among a large sample of transgender, nonbinary, and gender-diverse populations in Washington State, 2023. *Am J Public Health*. 2026;116(2):229–239.

Acceptance Date: October 9, 2025.

DOI: https://doi.org/10.2105/AJPH.2025.308312

ORCID iDs:

Adedotun Ogunbajo https://orcid.org/0000-0002-3074-6431

Teresa DeAtley https://orcid.org/0000-0002-2234-1629

Aaron Breslow https://orcid.org/0000-0003-2894-7485

Don Operario https://orcid.org/0000-0003-2467-5048

Rebecca L. Emery Tavernier https://orcid.org/0000-0002-9541-6791

CONTRIBUTORS

The authors contributed equally to the work.

ACKNOWLEDGMENTS

This study was funded by the University of Washington Center for AIDS Research (grant AI027757) and the University of Washington Behavioral Research Center for HIV (grant P30MH123248).

Note. The contents of this article are solely the responsibility of the authors and do not necessarily represent the official views of the funders.

CONFLICTS OF INTEREST

The authors have no conflicts of interest to disclose.

HUMAN PARTICIPANT PROTECTION

The Human Subject Division of the University of Washington's institutional review board approved all study procedures (no. STUDY00015878). All enrolled participants provided electronic informed consent and consent for publication.

REFERENCES

1. Patterson CJ, Riskind RG. To be a parent: issues in family formation among gay and lesbian adults. *J GLBT Fam Stud.* 2010;6(3):326–340. https://doi.org/10.1080/1550428X.2010.490902
2. Riskind RG, Patterson CJ. Parenting intentions and desires among childless lesbian, gay, and heterosexual individuals. *J Fam Psychol.* 2010; 24(1):78–81. https://doi.org/10.1037/a0017941
3. Mezzalira S, Della Casa V, Malmquist A, et al. Parenting desire and intention in the health trajectories of transgender and gender diverse people: a systematic review. *LGBTQ+ Fam.* 2024;1–21. https://doi.org/10.1080/27703371.2024.2427763
4. Kyweluk MA, Kirkley J, Grimstad F, Amato P, Downing J. Desire for genetically related children among transgender and gender-diverse patients seeking gender-affirming hormones. *F S Rep.* 2023;4(2):224–230. https://doi.org/10.1016/j.xfre.2023.04.004
5. Di Battista S, Shenkman G, Gato J, et al. Attitudes toward adoption by transgender adults. *LGBTQ+ Fam.* 2025;21(3):267–281. https://doi.org/10.1080/27703371.2024.2427768
6. Ducheny KM, Ehrbar RD. Family creation options for transgender and gender nonconforming people. *Psychol Sex Orientat Gend Divers.* 2016;3(2):173–179. https://doi.org/10.1037/sgd0000178
7. Johnson A, McClurg AB, Baldino J, Das R, Carey ET. Fertility preservation choices and decisional regret after gender-affirming surgery in transgender men or gender nonbinary persons. *F S Rep.* 2024;5(1):87–94. https://doi.org/10.1016/j.xfre.2023.12.002
8. Sevelius JM. Gender affirmation: a framework for conceptualizing risk behavior among transgender women of color. *Sex Roles.* 2013;68(11–12): 675–689. https://doi.org/10.1007/s11199-012-0216-5
9. Brown C. Exploring trans people's experiences of adoption and fostering in the United Kingdom: a qualitative study. *Int J Transgend Health.* 2021; 22(1–2):89–100. https://doi.org/10.1080/26895269.2020.1867396
10. Costa D. The influence of social capital on health issues among transgender and gender diverse people: a rapid review. *Science & Philosophy.* 2022;10(2): 109–131. https://doi.org/10.23756/sp.v10i2.934
11. Goldberg AE, Tornello S, Farr R, Smith JZ, Miranda L. Barriers to adoption and foster care and openness to child characteristics among transgender adults. *Child Youth Serv Rev.* 2020;109:104699. https://doi.org/10.1016/j.childyouth.2019.104699
12. Brown C, Rogers M. Removing gender barriers: promoting inclusion for trans and non-binary carers in fostering and adoption. *Child Fam Soc Work.* 2020;25(3):594–601. https://doi.org/10.1111/cfs.12731
13. Garborcauskas G, McCabe E, Boskey ER, Grimstad FW. Family building perspectives of assigned female at birth transgender and gender diverse adolescents seeking testosterone gender-affirming hormone therapy. *LGBT Health.* 2022;9(7):463–470. https://doi.org/10.1089/lgbt.2022.0004
14. Chen D, Berona J, Chan Y-M, et al. Psychosocial functioning in transgender youth after 2 years of hormones. *N Engl J Med.* 2023;388(3):240–250. https://doi.org/10.1056/NEJMoa2206297
15. Restar A, Jin H, Breslow A, et al. Legal gender marker and name change is associated with lower negative emotional response to gender-based mistreatment and improved mental health outcomes among trans populations. *SSM Popul Health.* 2020;11:100595. https://doi.org/10.1016/j.ssmph.2020.100595
16. Nixon L. The right to (trans) parent: a reproductive justice approach to reproductive rights, fertility, and family-building issues facing transgender people. *Wm Mary J Women Law.* 2013;20(1):72–103.
17. Katz-Wise SL, Ehrensaft D, Vetters R, Forcier M, Austin SB. Family functioning and mental health of transgender and gender-nonconforming youth in the trans teen and family narratives project. *J Sex Res.* 2018;55(4–5):582–590. https://doi.org/10.1080/00224499.2017.1415291
18. Movement Advancement Project. Parental recognition laws. 2025. Available at: https://www.lgbtmap.org/equality-maps/recognition/parenting. Accessed November 15, 2025.
19. Restar A, Minalga BJ, Quilantang MI, et al. Mapping community-engaged implementation strategies with transgender scientists, stakeholders, and trans-led community organizations. *Curr HIV/AIDS Rep.* 2023;20(3):160–169. https://doi.org/10.1007/s11904-023-00656-y
20. Restar A, Layland EK, Hughes L, et al. Antitrans policy environment and depression and anxiety symptoms in transgender and nonbinary adults. *JAMA Netw Open.* 2024;7(8):e2431306. https://doi.org/10.1001/jamanetworkopen.2024.31306
21. King WM, Gamarel KE. A scoping review examining social and legal gender affirmation and health among transgender populations. *Transgend Health.* 2021;6(1):5–22. https://doi.org/10.1089/trgh.2020.0025
22. Health Canada. The Household Food Security Survey Module (HFSSM). May 2, 2018. Available at: https://www.canada.ca/en/health-canada/services/food-nutrition/food-nutrition-surveillance/health-nutrition-surveys/canadian-community-health-survey-cchs/household-food-insecurity-canada-overview/household-food-security-survey-module-hfssm-health-nutrition-surveys-health-canada.html. Accessed November 15, 2025.
23. Akinwande MO, Dikko HG, Samson A. Variance inflation factor: a condition for the inclusion of suppressor variables in regression analysis. *Open J Stat.* 2015;5(7):754–767. https://doi.org/10.4236/ojs.2015.57075
24. Seelman KL, Colón-Diaz MJ, LeCroix RH, Xavier-Brier M, Kattari L. Transgender noninclusive healthcare and delaying care because of fear: connections to general health and mental health among transgender adults. *Transgend Health.* 2017;2(1):17–28. https://doi.org/10.1089/trgh.2016.0024
25. Sterling J, Garcia MM. Fertility preservation options for transgender individuals. *Transl Androl Urol.* 2020;9(suppl 2):S215–S226. https://doi.org/10.21037/tau.2019.09.28
26. Asseler J, de Nie I, van Rooij F, et al. Transgender persons' views on previous fertility decision-making and current infertility: a qualitative study. *Hum Reprod.* 2024;39(9):2032–2042. https://doi.org/10.1093/humrep/deae155
27. Nahata L, Curci MB, Quinn GP. Exploring fertility preservation intentions among transgender youth. *J Adolesc Health.* 2018;62(2):123–125. https://doi.org/10.1016/j.jadohealth.2017.11.288
28. Blakemore JK, Quinn GP, Fino ME. A discussion of options, outcomes, and future recommendations for fertility preservation for transmasculine individuals. *Urol Clin North Am.* 2019;46(4): 495–503. https://doi.org/10.1016/j.ucl.2019.07.014
29. Brehm M. The economics of adoption. In: Fenton-Glynn C, Lowe N, eds. *Research Handbook on Adoption Law.* Cheltenham, UK: Edward Elgar; 2023:58–77.
30. Cull MJ, Holroyd J. Gender-neutrality and family leave policies. In: LePore E, Lepore E, Anderson L, eds. *The Oxford Handbook of Applied Philosophy of Language.* Oxford, UK: Oxford University Press; 2024:364.
31. Hammoud Z. *Don't Leave Them Out: An International Comparative Analysis of Parental Leave Policies for Multiple Family Structures.* 2023. Available at: https://dspace.library.uvic.ca/server/api/core/bitstreams/af916395-5dfc-4745-9292-c5d818228e33/content. Accessed November 15, 2025.
32. Catalpa JM, McGuire JK. Family boundary ambiguity among transgender youth. *Fam Relat.* 2018;67(1): 88–103. https://doi.org/10.1111/fare.12304
33. Tornello SL, Riskind RG, Babić A. Transgender and gender non-binary parents' pathways to parenthood. *Psychol Sex Orientat Gend Divers.* 2019;6(2):232–241. https://doi.org/10.1037/sgd0000323
34. Hafford-Letchfield T, Cocker C, Rutter D, Tinarwo M, McCormack K, Manning R. What do we know about transgender parenting? Findings from a systematic review. *Health Soc Care Community.* 2019;27(5): 1111–1125. https://doi.org/10.1111/hsc.12759
35. Reisner SL, Radix A, Deutsch MB. Integrated and gender-affirming transgender clinical care and research. *J Acquir Immune Defic Syndr.* 2016; 72(suppl 3):S235–S242. https://doi.org/10.1097/QAI.0000000000001088

Structural Cissexism, Mental Health, and Unmet Health Care Needs Among Gender-Diverse Adolescents in the United States

Hyemin Lee, PhD, Tara R. Sullivan, Jessica R. Abramson, Peter S. McCauley, Ryan J. Watson, PhD, and Ethan H. Mereish, PhD

See also LGBTQ+ Well-Being and Joy, pp. 188–239.

AJPH February 2026, Vol. 116, No. 2

Objectives. To examine the associations between state-level structural cissexism and both mental health and unmet mental health care needs among a large national sample of gender-diverse adolescents (GDAs).

Methods. We measured structural cissexism by using a composite index of state-level indicators, including antitransgender laws and policies and explicit cissexist attitudes. Using participants' state identifiers, we linked this measure to individual-level mental health data from a subsample of 5658 GDAs (aged 13–18 years; mean age = 15.8 years; SD = 1.5) from the LGBTQ National Teen Survey conducted in 2022.

Results. GDAs in states with higher levels of structural cissexism reported greater depression and anxiety symptoms compared with those in states with lower levels. In addition, compared with GDAs in states with lower structural cissexism, those in states with higher structural cissexism were more likely to report unmet mental health care needs.

Conclusions. Our findings demonstrate significant associations between structural cissexism and mental health and health care utilization among GDAs. These results underscore the urgent need for transgender-affirming and protective policies and multidimensional and multilevel interventions across social environments to support GDA well-being and ensure equitable access to mental health services. (*Am J Public Health*. 2026;116(2):240–250. https://doi.org/10.2105/AJPH.2025.308313)

Gender-diverse adolescents (GDAs; e.g., transgender and nonbinary adolescents) report worse mental health outcomes compared with their cisgender peers,[1] potentially necessitating the need for and utilization of mental health care services.[2] Recent research indicates that GDAs not only experience greater mental health concerns, such as depressive symptoms and suicidal ideation, but also express higher willingness to seek help from counselors or therapists than cisgender adolescents.[3] Despite GDAs' mental health disparities and willingness toward accessing mental health care services, several factors, including discrimination within health care settings and lack of provider knowledge about transgender-specific needs, may impede access and use of such services when needed.[4,5]

Mental health disparities among GDAs have predominantly been attributed to individual-level experiences of cissexism,[6] which manifests in both interpersonal and intrapersonal forms.[7,8] Interpersonal cissexism includes active discrimination (e.g., harassment, rejection, or denial of services) and passive exclusion (e.g., assumptions of cisgender identity in everyday interactions). Intrapersonal cissexism involves internalized negative beliefs about one's gender identity and strategic identity concealment for safety. However, because not all forms of structural cissexism are readily apparent or consciously perceived by GDAs, research relying primarily on individual-level measures may systematically underestimate the full scope and impact of oppression on mental health outcomes. Moreover, this primary focus on individual-level experiences has resulted in a dearth of research examining how structural forms of cissexism affect GDAs' mental health, thereby limiting our understanding of the broader systemic forces contributing to these disparities.[6]

Structural cissexism is multidimensional and mutually informed by institutional laws, policies, social attitudes, and cultural norms that systematically restrict opportunities and resources for gender-diverse individuals,[9] including both explicitly discriminatory policies (e.g., bans on gender-affirming care) and systemic barriers (e.g., lack of transgender-inclusive health care coverage). In 2024, 701 antitransgender bills were introduced across the country, of which 207 specifically targeted GDAs in educational settings.[10] Alarmingly, an estimated 96 800 GDAs aged 13 to 17 years—nearly one third of the GDA population—live in states that enacted cissexist restrictions affecting their access to health care, sports participation, or school bathroom use in 2023.[11] Given these nationwide legislative attacks targeting gender-diverse populations and the substantial number of affected GDAs, understanding how structural cissexism shapes GDAs' mental health and health care experiences is essential for informing meaningful structural-level interventions.

Ecosocial theory[12]—which posits that social inequalities in health arise from the embodiment of complex and cumulative interactions between societal institutions, communities, and individuals—provides a framework for understanding how structural cissexism contributes to population-level health disparities among GDAs. Structurally cissexist policies and institutions facilitate societal invalidation and marginalization of GDAs, creating chronic stressors that become biologically embodied and manifest as poor mental health outcomes and unmet health care needs. Existing literature with primarily adult samples consistently demonstrates that structural cissexism is associated with greater psychological distress and mental health concerns,[13–19] but negatively associated with mental health care utilization.[20,21] Specifically regarding mental health care utilization, gender-diverse adults who reside in states with higher levels of structural cissexism were less likely to seek gender-affirming care services, including psychotherapy or counseling,[20,21] suggesting that transgender-inclusive and protective laws and policies may facilitate greater access to mental health care services. Moreover, states with higher levels of structural cissexism had restrictive state laws or policies that manifested in health care environments with fewer adolescent-focused mental health providers specializing in transgender-specific care,[22] further impeding GDAs' access to and utilization of mental health care.

While significant associations between structural cissexism and both mental health[13–19] and mental health care utilization[16,20,21] have been demonstrated, several knowledge gaps remain in this field. First, most studies have focused on gender-diverse adults, with only one known study examining GDAs,[17] particularly concerning given recent antitransgender legislation increasingly targeting transgender youths. Notably, Miller-Jacobs et al. examined associations between state-level policies and mental and behavioral health among transgender adolescents from 14 states.[17] Their analysis of 4 sexual and gender minority (SGM)–specific policies (e.g., antibullying laws, transgender student guidance) revealed protective associations between specific affirming policies and reduced depression and cigarette use. The current study extends this foundational work by expanding geographic scope beyond the 14-state limitation and developing a composite structural cissexism index that incorporates several laws and policies and social attitudes. Second, the assessment of structural cissexism has primarily relied on laws and policies related to gender-diverse individuals' rights. Whereas the presence of laws and policies provides more objective assessments of structural oppression, the assessment of social attitudes provides a lens into the cultural norms and customs of an environment that both shape and are shaped by such laws and policies.[9] Thus, to fully capture gender-diverse individuals' experiences of structural cissexism, measures should quantify both antitransgender laws and policies and cissexist attitudes.[23] Third, to our knowledge, no previous studies have examined the association between structural cissexism and unmet mental health care needs in the GDA population.

To address these critical gaps, we investigated the associations between structural cissexism and both depression and anxiety symptoms and unmet mental health care needs among GDAs. We assessed structural cissexism using publicly available data sets: (1) the Movement Advancement Project (MAP) policy tracking database,[24] which documents 45 state-level transgender-related laws or policies, and (2) Project Implicit's database,[25] which includes measures of explicit cissexist attitudes

AJPH February 2026, Vol. 116, No. 2

among thousands of respondents throughout the United States. Using both data sources and following recent methodological approaches in the field,[19,22,26] we developed a composite index that captures multiple components of structural cissexism, including antitransgender laws and policies and explicit cissexist attitudes. We hypothesized that GDAs in US states with higher structural cissexism would experience greater depression and anxiety symptoms and report more unmet mental health care needs than those in states with lower structural cissexism.

METHODS

We analyzed a subsample of GDAs (n = 5658) from the LGBTQ National Teen Survey of 17 578 SGM adolescents aged 13 to 18 years conducted in 2022. This nonprobability sample was recruited through multiple social media platforms and in-person advertising. Study graphics reached more than 1 million people on Facebook and Instagram, with community partners extending recruitment to Reddit, Discord, Twitch, and TikTok. Informed assent was obtained from all participants. Parental consent was waived, consistent with established practices in previous research involving SGM adolescents.[27] More detailed information has been described elsewhere.[28]

Individual-level data provided information on state of residence, mental health and health care outcomes, and demographic characteristics, which were merged with state-level structural cissexism measures. Of the 17 578 participants, 11 170 (63.5%) identified as gender diverse. Among GDA participants, missing values occurred as follows: state information (n = 3442; 30.8%), race and ethnicity (n = 14; 0.1%), sex assigned at birth (n = 47; 0.4%), depression and anxiety symptoms (n = 2009; 18.0%), and mental health care utilization (n = 494; 4.4%). The final analytic sample was 5658 participants for depression and anxiety analyses and 5164 participants for health care utilization analyses, representing all 50 states and the District of Columbia (DC).

Analysis of missingness patterns revealed systematic nonresponse among participants. Of the 2009 participants with incomplete 4-item Patient Health Questionnaire for Depression and Anxiety (PHQ-4) data, 1958 (97.5%) were missing all 4 PHQ-4 items. Among these participants, 1773 (90.6%) also had missing values for both mental health care utilization questions. As both the PHQ-4 and utilization items were located toward the end of the survey, this pattern suggests systematic rather than random missingness. The missingness likely reflects survey noncompletion or participant dropout rather than item-specific nonresponse. Given the systematic and extensive nature of the missingness pattern, we employed listwise deletion to avoid potentially biased estimates that could result from imputation models with insufficient information to reliably estimate missing values.

Measures

We measured structural cissexism using a composite index of state-level indicators and linked this measure to participants' individual mental health data using state identifiers.

Structural cissexism. To quantify structural cissexism across US states and the District of Columbia, we developed an index using state-level data from 2 sources: (1) antitransgender laws and policies from the MAP[24] and (2) explicit attitudes toward transgender people from Project Implicit.[25]

MAP is a nonprofit organization that tracks states' laws and policies specific to sexual orientation and gender identity across the United States.[24] As of March 2022, MAP included 45 state-level SGM-related laws and policies across 7 domains[24]:

1. relationship and parental recognition,
2. nondiscrimination,
3. religious exemptions,
4. youths,
5. health care,
6. criminal justice, and
7. identity documents.

Consistent with previous work,[19,22] we specifically used the comprehensive gender identity indicators from the MAP. We assigned scores to individual laws and policies in each US state and the District of Columbia as follows: −1 (restrictive), 0 (absent), and 1 (supportive). We summed scores for individual laws and policies across the 7 domains. Complete details on such laws and policies can be accessed through the MAP website,[24] though policies may have changed since March 2022.

Project Implicit is a web-based platform offering the Implicit Association Test and explicit measures of attitudes toward transgender people.[29] We incorporated indicators of state-level antitransgender explicit attitudes using data from Project Implicit, which have been administered since 2020 (pooled across years 2020–2022). Explicit attitudes were measured from thermometer items in which participants rated how warm or cold they felt toward cisgender and transgender people on a 0 (coldest) to 10 (warmest) scale. State-level aggregate scores were calculated by averaging individual ratings for cisgender and transgender people within each state. To reflect the comparative nature of regional attitudes scores, explicit attitudes were operationalized as a difference score computed at the state level.[30,31] Specifically, this difference score was calculated by subtracting the average cisgender rating from the average transgender rating. Of the 629 620 initial responses, 235 383 responses were included in the final analysis after removing those with missing state information (n = 379 960) and missing explicit attitudes data (n = 14 277).

Consistent with previous work,[19,22,26] we examined the psychometric properties of our state-level structural cissexism index by conducting an exploratory factor analysis on each state's MAP scores (7 domains included individually) and explicit attitudes toward transgender people. We leveraged factor analysis to minimize measurement error and enhance construct validity in structural stigma measurement, while recognizing high correlations among structural cissexism indicators (r = 0.53–0.77).[19,22,26] We reverse-coded all indicators where necessary to ensure that higher values indicated greater structural cissexism and then standardized. Following these steps, we conducted factor analysis on these indicators. The scree plot with parallel analysis suggested a 1-factor solution, with factor loadings ranging from 0.59 to 0.97 (Table A, available as a supplement to the online version of this article at https://ajph.org), explaining 69% of variance in state-level structural cissexism indicators. We computed model-generated, normally distributed factor scores for each state, with state-level structural cissexism being lowest in Oregon (−1.31) and highest in Alabama (1.83; Figure 1; Table B, available as a supplement to the online version of this article at https://ajph.org).

Depression and anxiety symptoms. Symptoms of depression and anxiety were assessed using the PHQ-4,[32] a 4-item screening scale in which participants rated the frequency of such symptoms over the past 2 weeks from 0 (not at all) to 3 (nearly every day). PHQ-4 sum scores ranged from 0 to 12, with good internal consistency (Cronbach $\alpha = 0.83$).

Mental health care utilization. We assessed mental health care utilization by using 2 questions: whether participants had received therapy or counseling services in the past 12 months, and if not, whether they wished they had. Response options for both questions were "Yes" or "No." Based on the combined responses to these 2 questions, we classified participants into 3 categories: (1) received care, (2) unmet mental health care needs (wished for but did not receive care), (3) neither wished for nor received care.

Demographic variables. Participants reported their age, race and ethnicity, sex assigned at birth, gender identity, and sexual orientation; survey questions and response categories are presented in Table C (available as a supplement to the online version of this article at https://ajph.org).

Analytic Plan

We conducted all statistical analyses using R version 4.3.1 (R Foundation for Statistical Computing, Vienna, Austria). For the analysis of health care utilization outcomes, we included 5164 GDA participants after excluding those with missing data on utilization questions (n = 494). Although participants were nested within states, we did not use multilevel models because of minimal clustering (intraclass correlation coefficients = 0.002–0.003). Instead, we calculated cluster-robust standard errors using the sandwich package in R[33,34] for linear regression models examining depression and anxiety symptoms and developed a custom implementation analyzing multinomial regression models for mental health care utilization.[35] This approach adjusted standard error estimates to account for potential within-state correlations.

In the adjusted models, we included age, race and ethnicity, sex assigned at birth, gender identity, and sexual orientation as covariates. These demographic variables are related to exposure to structural cissexism and independently impact mental health outcomes, thus meeting confounding criteria. For example, race and ethnicity shape structural cissexism exposure through residential segregation patterns rooted in legacies of White supremacy and intersectional experiences of racism and cissexism.[36] Sexual orientation may be associated with structural cissexism exposure through SGM community networks and geographic clustering in areas with varying levels of acceptance and resources.[37] There are also well-documented mental health inequities across each demographic category attributable to stigma, prejudice, and discrimination.[38] Therefore, they were conceptualized as potential confounders that could create spurious associations between structural cissexism and mental health outcomes if not controlled, consistent with established structural cissexism research.[13–21] Correlation analyses confirmed that these demographic characteristics show significant associations with mental health and health

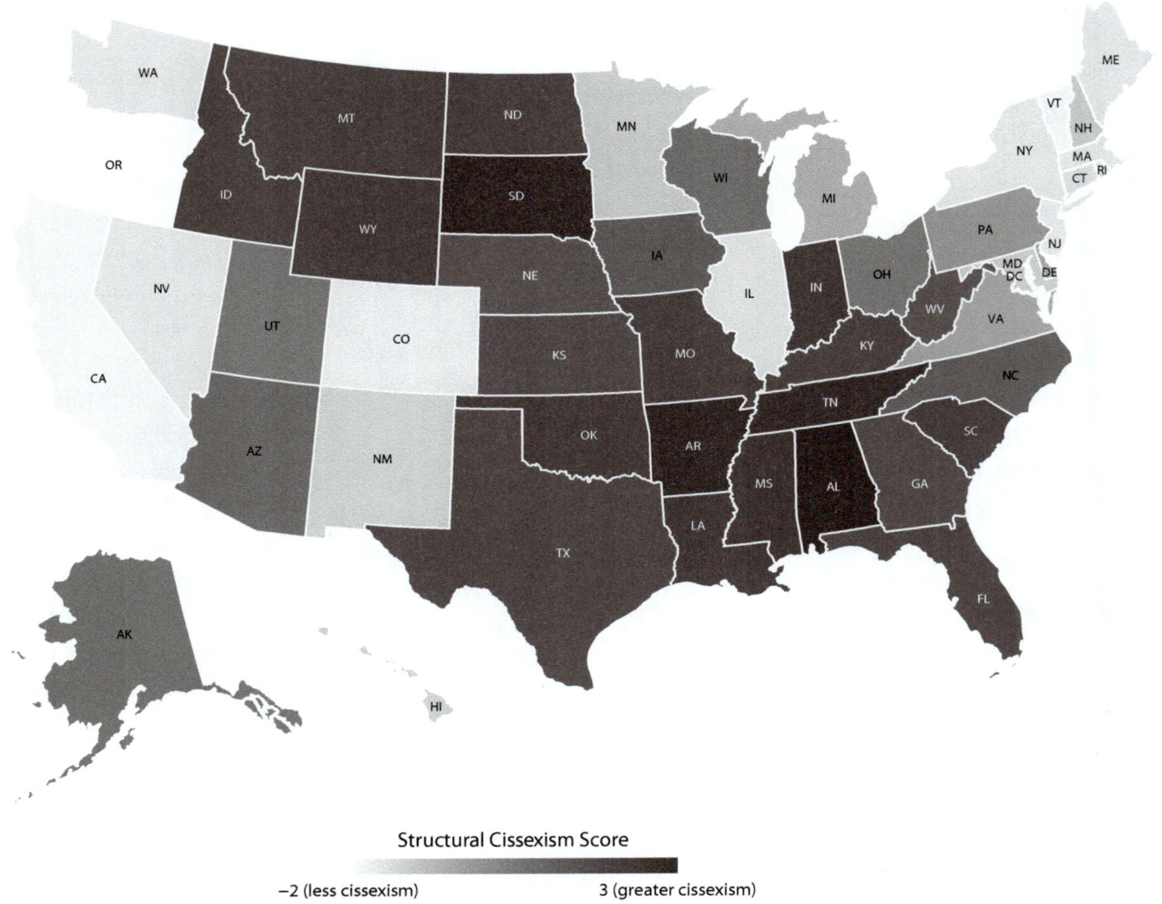

FIGURE 1— Structural Cissexism Factor Scores by State and District of Columbia Using State-Level Data From Movement Advancement Project (2022) and Project Implicit (2020–2022): United States

Note. Each state score is provided in Table B (available as a supplement to the online version of this article at https://ajph.org).

care outcomes (except for sexual orientation and its association with depression and anxiety symptoms), supporting their inclusion as confounders in our models. For multinomial regression models examining mental health care utilization, we also included the summed score of the PHQ-4 to adjust for mental health symptoms.

RESULTS

Of the 5658 GDAs included in our analysis, the mean age was 15.8 years (SD = 1.5), with the majority (59.8%) identifying as nonbinary or other gender identity (Table 1). We used the PHQ-4 to assess depression and anxiety symptoms, which had a mean score of 6.9 (SD = 3.3; median score = 6.0), indicating moderate symptoms.[32] Nearly 35% of the sample reported unmet mental health care needs.

Structural cissexism was significantly associated with depression and anxiety symptoms (adjusted $b = 0.11$; robust SE = 0.04; 95% confidence interval [CI] = 0.02, 0.20), even after adjusting for individual-level demographic characteristics (Table 2). Specifically, GDAs who lived in states with higher structural cissexism reported greater levels of depression and anxiety symptoms than those who lived in states with lower structural cissexism. To contextualize these findings, GDAs in states with high versus low structural cissexism have expected PHQ-4 scores of 7.05 and 6.83, respectively, demonstrating a 0.22-point difference that shifts individuals from the 46th to 55th percentile of depression and anxiety symptoms. This difference shows how state-level policies can meaningfully impact mental health outcomes at the population

AJPH February 2026, Vol. 116, No. 2

TABLE 1— Descriptive Statistics for Demographic Characteristics of the Gender-Diverse Adolescents: United States, LGBTQ National Teen Survey, 2022

	Full Sample (n = 5658), No. (%) or Mean ±SD
Age, y; range = 13–18 y	15.8 ±1.5
Race and ethnicity	
Non-Hispanic White	3786 (66.9)
Non-Hispanic Asian or Asian American	197 (3.5)
Non-Hispanic Black/African American	218 (3.9)
Hispanic/Latine	919 (16.2)
Non-Hispanic American Indian/Alaska Native/Pacific Islander	34 (0.6)
Non-Hispanic biracial/multiracial	465 (8.2)
Non-Hispanic other racial and ethnic minority	39 (0.7)
Sex assigned at birth	
Male	1472 (26.0)
Female	4167 (73.7)
Intersex	19 (0.3)
Gender identity	
Nonbinary	2543 (45.0)
Transgender boy	1634 (28.9)
Transgender girl	643 (11.4)
Other gender identity	838 (14.8)
Sexual orientation	
Gay or lesbian	1327 (23.5)
Bisexual	1380 (24.4)
Queer	747 (13.2)
Pansexual	969 (17.1)
Asexual	596 (10.5)
Other	639 (11.3)
Depression and anxiety symptoms (PHQ-4; range = 0–12)	6.9 ±3.3
Mental health care utilization[a]	
Received	3047 (59.0)
Unmet mental health care needs (wished for but not received)	1778 (34.4)
Neither wished for nor received	339 (6.6)

Note. PHQ-4 = 4-item Patient Health Questionnaire for Depression and Anxiety.
[a]Missing values in mental health care utilization = 494.

level through moving adolescents across clinically relevant thresholds.

Our multinomial regression analyses revealed a significant association between structural cissexism and mental health care utilization (Table 3). Specifically, GDAs who lived in states with higher structural cissexism had a greater likelihood of reporting unmet needs (adjusted odds ratio [AOR] = 1.10; 95% CI = 1.08, 1.13). We also found a significant association between structural cissexism and the "neither wished for nor received care" category when compared with the "received care" category (AOR = 0.95; 95% CI = 0.93, 0.97), indicating that GDAs in states with greater structural cissexism were less likely to report neither wishing for nor receiving care. To test the robustness of our composite structural cissexism index and whether each indicator independently contributes to outcomes, we conducted sensitivity analyses (1) performing multiple imputation analysis and (2) examining each MAP policy domain individually and the explicit cissexist attitudes indicator separately. These analyses showed consistent results in general, supporting the validity of our composite index (Tables 2 and 3).

DISCUSSION

Considering the exponential increase in antitransgender laws and policies across US states,[39] it is imperative to understand how such structurally cissexist restrictions may impact the health and well-being of GDAs. We developed a composite index of structural cissexism to examine the associations between structural cissexism, mental health, and unmet mental health care needs among GDAs. As hypothesized, our findings demonstrate positive associations between structural cissexism and depression and anxiety symptoms as well as unmet mental health care needs, such that those GDAs in states with higher structural cissexism reported greater depression and anxiety symptoms and unmet needs. These results are consistent with previous research that has theorized the harmful health impacts of antitransgender laws and policies, primarily among gender-diverse adults.[13–21] Our findings are among the first to examine the association between structural cissexism and its effects on GDAs' well-being, extending previous work by using a composite index of structural cissexism toward adolescent populations.

TABLE 2— Association Between Structural Cissexism and Depression and Anxiety Symptoms Among Gender-Diverse Adolescents: United States, LGBTQ National Teen Survey, 2022

Continuous Outcome	Adjusted Model, b (SE; 95% CI)
Main analysis	
Composite index: structural cissexism	0.11 (0.04; 0.02, 0.20)
Sensitivity analyses	
Analysis 1: multiple imputation analysis (n = 7667[a])	
Model 1. structural cissexism	0.09 (0.05; 0.00, 0.18)
Analysis 2: gender identity policy domain individually (Movement Advancement Project)	
Model 2-1. relationship and parental recognition	0.06 (0.05; −0.04, 0.15)
Model 2-2. nondiscrimination	0.04 (0.04; −0.04, 0.13)
Model 2-3. religious exemptions	0.06 (0.04; −0.02, 0.14)
Model 2-4. youths	0.11 (0.04; 0.03, 0.20)
Model 2-5. health care	0.13 (0.04; 0.04, 0.21)
Model 2-6. criminal justice	0.12 (0.04; 0.04, 0.21)
Model 2-7. identity documents	0.10 (0.05; 0.01, 0.19)
Analysis 3: attitudinal indicator separately (Project Implicit)	
Model 3. explicit cissexist attitudes	0.10 (0.04; 0.02, 0.18)

Note. CI = confidence interval. Each row under "Sensitivity analyses" represents a separate model. Analysis 1 used multiple imputation (1 model), analysis 2 examined each policy domain from the Movement Advancement Project individually (7 separate models), and analysis 3 examined the attitudinal indicator from Project Implicit as a standalone predictor (1 model). Standard errors are cluster-robust, clustered by state, for linear regression models. Covariates for adjusted models included age, race and ethnicity, sex assigned at birth, gender identity, and sexual orientation. For categorical covariates, reference groups were "non-Hispanic/Latine White" for race and ethnicity, "male" for sex assigned at birth, "nonbinary" for gender identity, and "gay or lesbian" for sexual orientation. Reference categories were selected based on sample size (i.e., non-Hispanic/Latine White for race and ethnicity, nonbinary for gender identity) and theoretical considerations (i.e., male for sex assigned at birth, gay or lesbian for sexual orientation). Additional analyses including caregiver's education level as a proxy for socioeconomic status showed similar patterns of results, although this variable was excluded from main analyses because of substantial missing data.
[a]Multiple imputation analysis was performed for outcome variables only (depression/anxiety symptoms and unmet mental health care needs) using structural cissexism, state of residence, age, race and ethnicity, sex assigned at birth, gender identity, and sexual orientation as auxiliary variables. Twenty imputed data sets were generated using the MICE package in R version 4.3.1 with 10 iterations, and results were pooled using Rubin's rules. Analysis included 7667 gender-diverse adolescents from 17 578 total participants, excluding those not identifying as gender diverse (n = 6408) and those with missing state (n = 3442), race and ethnicity (n = 14), or sex assigned at birth (n = 47) data.

The significant and positive associations between structural cissexism and depression and anxiety symptoms can be explained through multiple and interconnected pathways.[8,12] According to ecosocial theory[12] and the oppression-based stress framework,[6] cissexist laws and policies as well as hostile and unwelcoming environments for GDAs expose them to chronic stressors of cissexist discrimination. Previous work documents the associations between interpersonal cissexism (e.g., bullying, discrimination) and poorer mental health outcomes for GDAs,[40] as well as the potential for interpersonal cissexism to foster internalized cissexist attitudes.[7] This evidence suggests that structural cissexism operates across multiple socioecological levels, creating cascading effects that compound mental health risks for GDAs. In addition, these structural exposures become biologically embodied across critical developmental periods, manifesting as adverse mental health outcomes with potential long-term effects on mental health trajectories throughout the lifespan.

Our findings also indicate that GDAs in states with higher structural cissexism were more likely to report unmet mental health care needs, aligning with ecosocial theory[12] in suggesting how structural cissexism creates cascading barriers to health care access. Many cissexist bills have been deliberately introduced and formalized into laws across the United States that specifically limit access to transgender-affirming care, particularly for youths. Relatedly, previous research has demonstrated that states with more cissexist laws and policies have fewer transgender-specific adolescent mental health providers available.[22] Such provider shortage has been identified as a significant predictor of unmet mental health care needs among sexual-minority adolescents.[41] Beyond direct policy restrictions, overall cissexist environments may undermine familial support and acceptance, making it unsafe for GDAs to seek mental health care services because of risks of being outed, denied service, or harassed. This demonstrates how structural cissexism becomes embodied through both institutional and interpersonal barriers, ultimately limiting GDAs' ability to access supportive care.

Collectively, our findings underscore the importance of further research that examines structural cissexism and its impact on GDAs' health and health care

TABLE 3— Association Between Structural Cissexism and Mental Health Care Utilization Among Gender-Diverse Adolescents: United States, LGBTQ National Teen Survey, 2022

Categorical Outcome	Adjusted Model, OR (95% CI)
Unmet mental health care needs (vs received)	
Main analysis, composite index: structural cissexism	1.10 (1.08, 1.13)
Sensitivity analysis 1: multiple imputation analysis (n = 7667[a])	
Model 1. structural cissexism	1.06 (1.03, 1.10)
Sensitivity analysis 2: gender identity policy domain individually (Movement Advancement Project)	
Model 2-1. relationship and parental recognition	1.09 (1.07, 1.11)
Model 2-2. nondiscrimination	1.09 (1.06, 1.11)
Model 2-3. religious exemptions	1.09 (1.07, 1.12)
Model 2-4. youths	1.10 (1.08, 1.13)
Model 2-5. health care	1.10 (1.08, 1.12)
Model 2-6. criminal justice	1.07 (1.05, 1.09)
Model 2-7. identity documents	1.08 (1.06, 1.11)
Sensitivity analysis 3: attitudinal indicator separately (Project Implicit)	
Model 3. explicit cissexist attitudes	1.08 (1.06, 1.10)
Neither wished for nor received (vs received)	
Main analysis, composite index: structural cissexism	0.95 (0.93, 0.97)
Sensitivity analysis 1: multiple imputation analysis (n = 7667[a])	
Model 1. structural cissexism	1.02 (0.96, 1.08)
Sensitivity analysis 2: gender identity policy domain individually (Movement Advancement Project)	
Model 2-1. relationship and parental recognition	1.01 (0.99, 1.04)
Model 2-2. nondiscrimination	0.95 (0.93, 0.97)
Model 2-3. religious exemptions	0.98 (0.96, 1.00)
Model 2-4. youths	0.97 (0.95, 0.99)
Model 2-5. health care	0.98 (0.96, 1.00)
Model 2-6. criminal justice	0.94 (0.92, 0.96)
Model 2-7. identity documents	0.98 (0.96, 1.00)
Sensitivity analysis 3: attitudinal indicator separately (Project Implicit)	
Model 3. explicit cissexist attitudes	0.90 (0.88, 0.92)

Note. CI = confidence interval; OR = odds ratio. Each model under sensitivity analysis 1, 2, and 3 represents a separate model. Sensitivity analysis 1 used multiple imputation (1 model), analysis 2 examined each policy domain from the Movement Advancement Project individually (7 separate models), and analysis 3 examined the attitudinal indicator from Project Implicit as a standalone predictor (1 model). Standard errors are cluster-robust, clustered by state, for multinomial logistic regression models. Covariates for adjusted models included age, race and ethnicity, sex assigned at birth, gender identity, sexual orientation, and the summed score of the 4-item Patient Health Questionnaire for Depression and Anxiety. For categorical covariates, reference groups were "non-Hispanic/Latine White" for race and ethnicity, "male" for sex assigned at birth, "nonbinary" for gender identity, and "gay or lesbian" for sexual orientation. Reference categories were selected based on sample size (i.e., non-Hispanic/Latine White for race and ethnicity, nonbinary for gender identity) and theoretical considerations (i.e., male for sex assigned at birth, gay or lesbian for sexual orientation). Additional analyses including caregiver's education level as a proxy for socioeconomic status showed similar patterns of results, although this variable was excluded from main analyses because of substantial missing data.
[a]Multiple imputation analysis was performed for outcome variables only (depression/anxiety symptoms and unmet mental health care needs) using structural cissexism, state of residence, age, race and ethnicity, sex assigned at birth, gender identity, and sexual orientation as auxiliary variables. Twenty imputed data sets were generated using the MICE package in R version 4.3.1 with 10 iterations, and results were pooled using Rubin's rules. Analysis included 7667 gender-diverse adolescents from 17 578 total participants, excluding those not identifying as gender diverse (n = 6408) and those with missing state (n = 3442), race and ethnicity (n = 14), or sex assigned at birth (n = 47) data.

utilization. To the best of our knowledge, only 1 other study has examined the health impacts tied to structural cissexism, using antitransgender laws and policies individually, among GDAs.[17] From a life course perspective, adolescence is a critical developmental period marked by rapid changes in social, physical, and cognitive development, making it an optimal time to examine how ontogenetic and sociohistorical time intersect to shape mental health symptomatology.[42,43] Exposure to structural cissexism may accumulate over time alongside exposures to other oppression-based stressors (e.g., bias-based harassment). This accumulation has the potential to deplete GDAs' preemptive coping resources and contribute to deleterious long-term effects on mental health during adulthood.[44] Critically, laws and policies, social attitudes, and cultural norms that contribute to structural cissexism are dynamic,[23] requiring longitudinal designs to capture how these changes in social, political, and legal environments over time impact GDAs' long-term health.

Limitations

Several limitations should be considered when interpreting our results. First, we used a nonprobability subsample of GDAs from a national survey, which limits the generalizability of our findings and potentially biases results toward those able to access the survey, those comfortable disclosing their gender identity, those with increased mental health symptomatology, and those with issues in accessing health care. Also, the systematic pattern of missingness, particularly the co-occurrence of missing PHQ-4 and health care utilization data, may limit generalizability given the observed differences in sociodemographic characteristics between included and excluded participants (Table D, available as a supplement to the online version of this article at https://ajph.org).

Second, causal inference is limited by our cross-sectional study design. In addition, while migration patterns among gender-diverse populations may introduce selection bias, this concern is likely reduced in our adolescent sample given their limited autonomy to relocate compared with adults. Third, while combining multiple indicators strengthened our measurement of structural cissexism, the data sources had different time frames (MAP from 2022 and Project Implicit pooled across 2020–2022), which may not accurately capture potential changes in attitudes over time. Fourth, our study has measurement limitations including the brief PHQ-4 assessment and the unmet needs measure (limited to therapy and counseling services and not capturing other dimensions of utilization barriers).

Despite these limitations, our study has notable strengths. We generated a composite index of structural cissexism, which included both antitransgender laws and policies and explicit cissexist attitudes, using publicly available data sets. This approach offers a deeper understanding of how structural cissexism—encompassing institutional laws, policies, and attitudes—impacts GDAs' mental health and health care utilization. In addition, our large, national, and geographically diverse sample allows broader conclusions about the impacts of structural cissexism on the lives of GDAs.

Conclusions and Policy Implications

Our novel findings underscore significant associations between state-level structural cissexism and both mental health symptoms and unmet mental health care needs among GDAs. As antitransgender legislation proliferates across the United States, these results highlight the urgent need for protective laws and policies and interventions to support GDAs' mental health and ensure equitable access to mental health care services. The downstream impacts of structural cissexism could be mitigated through the implementation of protective and affirming policies for GDAs. Multidimensional and multilevel approaches across social environments, such as antitransgender bullying policies in schools and initiatives to increase transgender-affirming clinician availability, are essential to counter structural cissexism and its embodied impacts on GDAs' mental health and health care accessibility. At the practice level, health care providers should recognize the structural challenges GDAs face and implement inclusive strategies (e.g., creating transgender-affirming clinical environments) to support their mental health and health care needs. Future research should prioritize multidimensional approaches to developing and validating measures of structural cissexism.[23] In addition, researchers should examine how structural cissexism impacts GDAs' mental health and health care utilization through an intersectional lens, exploring how it interacts with other forms of structural oppression and demographic characteristics. AJPH

ABOUT THE AUTHORS

Hyemin Lee was with the Lavender Lab, Department of Psychology, University of Maryland, College Park, at the time of this study. Tara R. Sullivan, Jessica R. Abramson, and Ethan H. Mereish are with the Lavender Lab, Department of Psychology, University of Maryland. Peter S. McCauley and Ryan J. Watson are with the Department of Human Development & Family Sciences, University of Connecticut, Storrs.

CORRESPONDENCE

Correspondence should be sent to Hyemin Lee, Department of Health and Exercise Science, University of Oklahoma, 1401 Asp Ave, Norman, OK 73019 (e-mail: hyemin.lee@ou.edu). Reprints can be ordered at https://www.ajph.org by clicking the "Reprints" link.

PUBLICATION INFORMATION

Full Citation: Lee H, Sullivan TR, Abramson JR, McCauley PS, Watson RJ, Mereish EH. Structural cissexism, mental health, and unmet health care needs among gender-diverse adolescents in the United States. *Am J Public Health*. 2026;116(2): 240–250.

Acceptance Date: October 9, 2025.

DOI: https://doi.org/10.2105/AJPH.2025.308313

ORCID iDs:

Hyemin Lee https://orcid.org/0000-0001-9257-6434

Tara R. Sullivan https://orcid.org/0000-0002-4230-0082

Jessica R. Abramson https://orcid.org/0000-0003-0622-7989

Peter S. McCauley https://orcid.org/0000-0001-8400-7311

Ryan J. Watson https://orcid.org/0000-0001-7824-7714

Ethan H. Mereish https://orcid.org/0000-0003-4655-0836

CONTRIBUTORS

H. Lee led the study's conceptualization and design, conducted formal analysis, interpreted the data, and took the lead in drafting and revising the article. T. R. Sullivan, J. R. Abramson, and P. S. McCauley contributed to data interpretation and participated in drafting and revising the article. R. J. Watson oversaw data collection and investigation and contributed to the article revision. E. H. Mereish played a key role in the study's conceptualization and design, contributed to data interpretation, and critically revised the article. All authors have reviewed and approved the final version of this article.

ACKNOWLEDGMENTS

This work was supported by the National Institute on Alcohol Abuse and Alcoholism (R01AA029989; PI: E. H. Mereish) and National Institute on Drug Abuse (K01DA047918; PI: R. J. Watson). Financial support was provided by the University of Oklahoma's Research Publication Subvention Funding Program.

CONFLICTS OF INTEREST

The authors declare no conflicts of interest.

HUMAN PARTICIPANT PROTECTION

All procedures were approved by the University of Connecticut's institutional review board.

REFERENCES

1. Wittlin NM, Kuper LE, Olson KR. Mental health of transgender and gender diverse youth. *Annu Rev Clin Psychol*. 2023;19(1):207–232. https://doi.org/10.1146/annurev-clinpsy-072220-020326
2. Mojtabai R, Olfson M. National trends in mental health care for US adolescents. *JAMA Psychiatry*. 2020;77(7):703–714. https://doi.org/10.1001/jamapsychiatry.2020.0279
3. Lucas R, Geierstanger S, Soleimanpour S. Mental health needs, barriers, and receipt of care among transgender and nonbinary adolescents. *J Adolesc Health*. 2024;75(2):267–274. https://doi.org/10.1016/j.jadohealth.2024.03.009
4. Henderson ER, Goldbach JT, Blosnich JR. Social determinants of sexual and gender minority mental health. *Curr Treat Options Psych*. 2022; 9(3):229–245. https://doi.org/10.1007/s40501-022-00269-z
5. Rees SN, Crowe M, Harris S. The lesbian, gay, bisexual and transgender communities' mental health care needs and experiences of mental health services: an integrative review of qualitative studies. *J Psychiatr Ment Health Nurs*. 2021; 28(4):578–589. https://doi.org/10.1111/jpm.12720
6. Mereish EH. Oppression-based stress and alcohol inequities among sexual and gender minority people: an intersectional multilevel framework. *Alcohol Res*. 2024;44(1):05. https://doi.org/10.35946/arcr.v44.1.05
7. Testa RJ, Habarth J, Peta J, Balsam K, Bockting W. Development of the Gender Minority Stress and Resilience Measure. *Psychol Sex Orientat Gend Divers*. 2015;2(1):65–77. https://doi.org/10.1037/sgd0000081
8. White Hughto JM, Reisner SL, Pachankis JE. Transgender stigma and health: a critical review of stigma determinants, mechanisms, and interventions. *Soc Sci Med*. 2015;147:222–231. https://doi.org/10.1016/j.socscimed.2015.11.010
9. Hatzenbuehler ML. Structural stigma: research evidence and implications for psychological science. *Am Psychol*. 2016;71(8):742–751. https://doi.org/10.1037/amp0000068
10. Trans Legislation Tracker. 2024 anti-trans legislation. 2024. Available at: https://translegislation.com/bills/2024. Accessed July 10, 2025.
11. Mallory C, Redfield E. The impact of 2023 legislation on transgender youth. Los Angeles, CA: Williams Institute, UCLA School of Law; 2023.
12. Krieger N. Theories for social epidemiology in the 21st century: an ecosocial perspective. *Int J Epidemiol*. 2001;30(4):668–677. https://doi.org/10.1093/ije/30.4.668
13. Blosnich JR, Marsiglio MC, Gao S, et al. Mental health of transgender veterans in US states with and without discrimination and hate crime legal protection. *Am J Public Health*. 2016;106(3): 534–540. https://doi.org/10.2105/AJPH.2015.302981
14. Drakeford L. Correctional policy and attempted suicide among transgender individuals. *J Correct Health Care*. 2018;24(2):171–182. https://doi.org/10.1177/1078345818764110
15. Du Bois SN, Yoder W, Guy AA, Manser K, Ramos S. Examining associations between state-level transgender policies and transgender health. *Transgend Health*. 2018;3(1):220–224. https://doi.org/10.1089/trgh.2018.0031
16. McDowell A, Raifman J, Progovac AM, Rose S. Association of nondiscrimination policies with mental health among gender minority individuals. *JAMA Psychiatry*. 2020;77(9):952–958. https://doi.org/10.1001/jamapsychiatry.2020.0770
17. Miller-Jacobs C, Operario D, Hughto JMW. State-level policies and health outcomes in US transgender adolescents: findings from the 2019 Youth Risk Behavior Survey. *LGBT Health*. 2023; 10(6):447–455. https://doi.org/10.1089/lgbt.2022.0247
18. Perez-Brumer A, Hatzenbuehler ML, Oldenburg CE, Bockting W. Individual- and structural-level risk factors for suicide attempts among transgender adults. *Behav Med*. 2015;41(3):164–171. https://doi.org/10.1080/08964289.2015.1028322
19. Price MA, Hollinsaid NL, McKetta S, Mellen EJ, Rakhilin M. Structural transphobia is associated with psychological distress and suicidality in a large national sample of transgender adults. *Soc Psychiatry Psychiatr Epidemiol*. 2024;59(2): 285–294. https://doi.org/10.1007/s00127-023-02482-4
20. Goldenberg T, Reisner SL, Harper GW, Gamarel KE, Stephenson R. State-level transgender-specific policies, race/ethnicity, and use of medical gender affirmation services among transgender and other gender-diverse people in the United States. *Milbank Q*. 2020;98(3):802–846. https://doi.org/10.1111/1468-0009.12467
21. Falck F, Bränström R. The significance of structural stigma towards transgender people in health care encounters across Europe: health care access, gender identity disclosure, and discrimination in health care as a function of national legislation and public attitudes. *BMC Public Health*. 2023;23(1):1031. https://doi.org/10.1186/s12889-023-15856-9
22. Hollinsaid NL, Price MA, Hatzenbuehler ML. Transgender-specific adolescent mental health provider availability is substantially lower in states with more restrictive policies. *J Clin Child Adolesc Psychol*. 2024;53(5):828–839. https://doi.org/10.1080/15374416.2022.2140433
23. Zubizarreta D, Trinh M-H, Reisner SL. Quantitative approaches to measuring structural cisgenderism. *Soc Sci Med*. 2024;340:116437. https://doi.org/10.1016/j.socscimed.2023.116437
24. Movement Advancement Project. Equality Maps: Snapshot: LGBTQ Equality By State. Available at: https://www.mapresearch.org/equality-maps. Accessed July 10, 2025.
25. Axt JR, Conway MA, Westgate EC, Buttrick NR. Implicit transgender attitudes independently predict beliefs about gender and transgender people. *Pers Soc Psychol Bull*. 2021;47(2): 257–274. https://doi.org/10.1177/0146167220921065
26. Lattanner MR, Ford J, Bo N, et al. A contextual approach to the psychological study of identity concealment: examining direct, interactive, and indirect effects of structural stigma on concealment motivation across proximal and distal geographic levels. *Psychol Sci*. 2021;32(10):1684–1696. https://doi.org/10.1177/09567976211018624
27. Mustanski B, Macapagal K, Matson M, Saber R. Evidence-based recommendations for ethical research practices with sexual and gender minority adolescents. Chicago, IL: Institute for Sexual and Gender Minority Health and Wellbeing, Northwestern University; 2023.
28. Watson RJ, Caba AE, Lawrence SE, et al. Examining mental health and bullying concerns at the intersection of sexuality, gender, race, and ethnicity among a national sample of sexual and gender diverse youth. *LGBT Health*. 2024;11(1): 20–27. https://doi.org/10.1089/lgbt.2023.0072
29. Charlesworth TE, Navon M, Rabinovich Y, Lofaro N, Kurdi B. The Project Implicit international dataset: measuring implicit and explicit social group attitudes and stereotypes across 34 countries (2009–2019). *Behav Res Methods*. 2023;55(3): 1413–1440. https://doi.org/10.3758/s13428-022-01851-2

30. Ofosu EK, Chambers MK, Chen JM, Hehman E. Same-sex marriage legalization associated with reduced implicit and explicit antigay bias. *Proc Natl Acad Sci U S A.* 2019;116(18):8846–8851. https://doi.org/10.1073/pnas.1806000116

31. Snyder JS, Henry P. Regional measures of sexual-orientation bias predict where same-gender couples live. *Psychol Sci.* 2023;34(7):794–808. https://doi.org/10.1177/09567976231173903

32. Kroenke K, Spitzer RL, Williams JB, Löwe B. An ultra-brief screening scale for anxiety and depression: the PHQ–4. *Psychosomatics.* 2009; 50(6):613–621. https://doi.org/10.1176/appi.psy.50.6.613

33. Zeileis A, Köll S, Graham N. Various versatile variances: an object-oriented implementation of clustered covariances in R. *J Stat Soft.* 2020; 95(1):1–36. https://doi.org/10.18637/jss.v095.i01

34. Zeileis A. Econometric computing with HC and HAC covariance matrix estimators. *J Stat Soft.* 2004;11(10):1–17. https://doi.org/10.18637/jss.v011.i10

35. Cameron AC, Miller DL. A practitioner's guide to cluster-robust inference. *J Hum Resour.* 2015;50(2): 317–372. https://doi.org/10.3368/jhr.50.2.317

36. Sumerau JE, Denise EJ. Obscuring oppression: racism, cissexism, and the persistence of social inequality. *Sociol Race Ethn (Thousand Oaks).* 2018; 4(3):322–337. https://doi.org/10.1177/2332649218755179

37. Paceley MS, Dikitsas ZA, Greenwood E, et al. The perceived health implications of policies and rhetoric targeting transgender and gender diverse youth: a community-based qualitative study. *Transgend Health.* 2023;8(1):100–103. https://doi.org/10.1089/trgh.2021.0125

38. Schwartz S, Meyer IH. Mental health disparities research: the impact of within and between group analyses on tests of social stress hypotheses. *Soc Sci Med.* 2010;70(8):1111–1118. https://doi.org/10.1016/j.socscimed.2009.11.032

39. Trans Legislation Tracker. Tracking the rise of anti-trans bills in the US. 2024. Available at: https://translegislation.com/learn. Accessed July 10, 2025.

40. Tankersley AP, Grafsky EL, Dike J, Jones RT. Risk and resilience factors for mental health among transgender and gender nonconforming (TGNC) youth: a systematic review. *Clin Child Fam Psychol Rev.* 2021;24(2):183–206. https://doi.org/10.1007/s10567-021-00344-6

41. Roulston C, McKetta S, Price M, Fox KR, Schleider JL. Structural correlates of mental health support access among sexual minority youth of color during COVID-19. *J Clin Child Adolesc Psychol.* 2023;52(5):649–658. https://doi.org/10.1080/15374416.2022.2034633

42. Fish JN. Future directions in understanding and addressing mental health among LGBTQ youth. *J Clin Child Adolesc Psychol.* 2020;49(6):943–956. https://doi.org/10.1080/15374416.2020.1815207

43. Russell ST, Fish JN. Sexual minority youth, social change, and health: a developmental collision. *Res Hum Dev.* 2019;16(1):5–20. https://doi.org/10.1080/15427609.2018.1537772

44. Hatzenbuehler ML. How does sexual minority stigma "get under the skin"? A psychological mediation framework. *Psychol Bull.* 2009;135(5): 707–730. https://doi.org/10.1037/a0016441

Evaluation of a Novel Data Source for National Influenza Surveillance: Influenza Hospitalization Data in the National Healthcare Safety Network, United States, September 2021–April 2024

Aaron M. Frutos, PhD, Shunte Moon, PhD, Alison M. Binder, MS, Andrea J. Cool, MPH, Kingsley Iyawe, MS, Trevor Thompson, Margaret A. Dudeck, MPH, Catherine H. Bozio, PhD, Mark W. Tenforde, MD, PhD, Matthew Biggerstaff, ScD, MPH, and Kelsey M. Sumner, PhD, MSPH

See also xxxx.

Objectives. To evaluate the completeness and utility of influenza hospital data reported to the Centers for Disease Control and Prevention's National Healthcare Safety Network (NHSN) from September 2021 to April 2024.

Methods. Acute care and critical access hospitals in the United States reported daily numbers of new hospital admissions of patients with laboratory-confirmed influenza to NHSN during voluntary and mandatory reporting periods. To evaluate the completeness of data reported to NHSN, we compared the number of influenza hospital admissions reported to NHSN with data reported to the Influenza Hospitalization Surveillance Network (FluSurv-NET) among 13 states and overlapping counties reporting to both systems from September 2021 to April 2024.

Results. During voluntary reporting, about 77% of US hospitals reported daily influenza hospital admission counts to NHSN; during mandatory reporting, this increased to a mean of 94%. These data were highly correlated ($r = 0.978$; 95% confidence interval = 0.968, 0.985; $P < .001$) with numbers from FluSurv-NET and in most states (r range = 0.861–0.988) within overlapping surveillance areas.

Conclusions. Influenza hospital admissions reported to NHSN demonstrate high levels of complete reporting; overall counts are highly correlated with a high-quality, long-standing influenza hospitalization surveillance system. (*Am J Public Health*. 2026;116(2):251–255. https://doi.org/10.2105/AJPH.2025.308282)

AJPH February 2026, Vol. 116, No. 2

The US Centers for Disease Control and Prevention (CDC) maintains year-round influenza surveillance to inform influenza control and prevention efforts.[1] To complement current surveillance and better understand the COVID-19 pandemic's impact on the US health care system, all acute care and critical access hospitals were required by the Centers for Medicare and Medicaid Services (CMS) Conditions of Participation to report health care utilization and capacity and COVID-19 hospital admissions from September 2020 through April 2024[2]; this created the nation's most comprehensive system for identifying emerging infectious threats, encompassing 6000 acute care hospitals in all US states and territories.[3] This system was leveraged for nationwide influenza hospitalization surveillance when optional influenza variables were added to the data collection in October 2020. Since then, there have been periods of voluntary and mandatory reporting of influenza variables based on influenza virus seasonality, operational capacity, and shifting public health priorities. Data collection is currently facilitated through CDC's National Healthcare Safety Network (NHSN; Supplemental Methods; Appendix Table A, available as a supplement to the online version of this article at https://ajph.org).[3]

METHODS

We evaluated the completeness and public health response utility of the influenza hospital admission data reported to NHSN during periods of voluntary and mandatory reporting. We examined data from September 2021 to April 2024 and compared it with data from the Influenza Hospitalization Surveillance Network (FluSurv-NET), a multisite, population-based influenza hospitalization surveillance system.[4]

Influenza hospital admissions in NHSN are defined as the previous day's new hospital admissions with laboratory-confirmed influenza virus infection within 14 days before or during hospitalization. From September 2021 to February 1, 2022, weekly influenza hospital admission reporting was voluntary with mandatory reporting beginning February 2, 2022. To evaluate data completeness, we calculated the weekly proportion of facilities reporting influenza hospital admissions by comparing the number of days of reported data by facility to the number of days of data that should have been reported for all facilities.

To explore if influenza hospital admissions in NHSN correlate with a long-standing, active, population-based influenza hospital surveillance system, we compared hospital admissions reported to NHSN with FluSurv-NET for counties represented in both systems for all 3 seasons (select counties in California, Colorado, Connecticut, Georgia, Maryland, Michigan, Minnesota, New Mexico, New York, Ohio, Oregon, Tennessee, and Utah), which covers approximately 9% of the US population. Briefly, FluSurv-NET conducts population-based surveillance for laboratory-confirmed influenza hospitalizations (including observations or emergency department encounters ≥ 24 hours or hospital transfers) in persons of all ages; trained surveillance staff review medical records to verify that patients meet the case definition. Because NHSN has near-real-time reporting of influenza hospital admissions from all US states and territories instead of a subset, we evaluated if the quick and broad capture of NHSN data were comparable in accuracy to FluSurv-NET, which represents only 9% of the country. FluSurv-NET was chosen for comparison with NHSN over influenza-like illness–based surveillance systems because of its requirement for laboratory confirmation of influenza infections, which is important with the emergence of COVID-19. Additional details are available in the Appendix (Supplemental Methods, Table A).

We aggregated daily data from September 2021 to April 2024 to weekly total admissions counts. We first calculated a Pearson correlation coefficient comparing hospital admissions for each week between NHSN and FluSurv-NET nationally and by state. Facilities not reporting influenza hospitalizations to NHSN were excluded from that week's influenza hospitalization count. We compared the national seasonal peaks of hospitalizations. We performed statistical analyses in R version 4.4.0 (R Foundation for Statistical Computing, Vienna, Austria).

RESULTS

From September 2021 to April 2024, there were 536 405 laboratory-confirmed influenza hospitalizations reported to NHSN from more than 5000 hospitals in all states, the District of Columbia, and 5 US territories. Before the mandatory reporting requirement began on February 2, 2022, 11% to 25%, with a mean of 22.7%, of facilities did not report daily influenza hospital admissions per week (Appendix Figure A); in 8 states, more than 50% of facilities did not report daily influenza hospitalizations (Appendix Figure B) per week; following February 2, 2022, when reporting was required, only 6% of facilities, on average, did not report daily influenza hospital admissions per week.

From February 2022 to April 2024, influenza hospital admissions in overlapping counties in NHSN and FluSurv-NET were highly correlated ($r = 0.978$; 95% confidence interval = 0.968, 0.985; $P < .001$; Figure 1 and Appendix Figure C). When we examined hospital admissions by state, we found admission counts reported to NHSN and FluSurv-NET were similar in most states; correlation coefficients ranged from 0.861 to 0.990 with the greatest difference between NHSN and FluSurv-NET occurring around the seasonal peaks for influenza activity (Appendix Figure D). When we compared these state-specific seasonal peaks across the 3 seasons (39 peaks, 1 peak for each of the 13 states per season), 29 out of 39 (74%) of the peaks were higher in FluSurv-NET than in NHSN. For 31 out of 39 (79%) of the state-specific seasonal peaks, the peaks in NHSN and FluSurv-NET occurred within 7 days of each other.

DISCUSSION

Influenza hospitalization data provide insights into the burden of influenza on hospitals and resource capacity. NHSN is the first system to provide complete

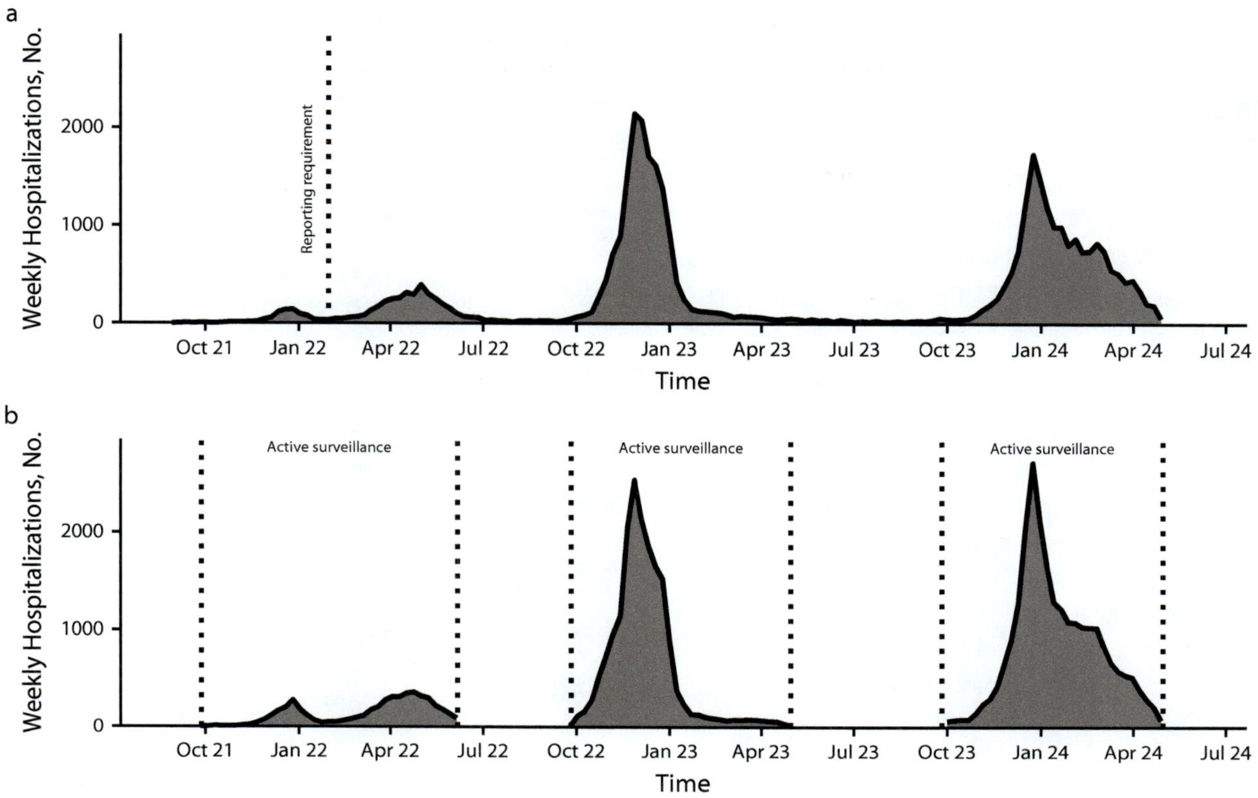

FIGURE 1— Weekly Laboratory-Confirmed Influenza Hospitalizations Within Overlapping Counties Reported to (a) the National Healthcare Safety Network and (b) FluSurv-NET: United States, September 2021–April 2024

Note. FluSurv-NET = Influenza Hospitalization Surveillance Network. Mandatory influenza hospitalization reporting for NHSN restarted on February 2, 2022. FluSurv-NET active surveillance during this period was October 1, 2021, to June 11, 2022; October 1, 2022, to April 30, 2023; and October 1, 2023, to April 30, 2024. Overlapping counties are from California, Colorado, Connecticut, Georgia, Maryland, Michigan, Minnesota, New Mexico, New York, Ohio, Oregon, Tennessee, and Utah. The correlation between NHSN and FluSurv-NET weekly hospitalizations (Pearson $r = 0.978$) can be seen in Appendix Figure C, available as a supplement to the online version of this article at https://www.ajph.org.

US national and state-level influenza-associated hospitalizations in near real time. These NHSN data are well correlated with a long-standing, high-quality active hospitalization surveillance system. We found that incident influenza hospital admission counts reported to NHSN were similar to those reported in FluSurv-NET within most overlapping geographic regions. Data missingness in NHSN was low during the mandatory reporting period.

These findings highlight the ability of NHSN to accurately capture real-time information on influenza hospitalizations at the national and state level, complementing other influenza surveillance systems such as FluSurv-NET. NHSN includes data from all hospitals registered with CMS across the United States and its territories to monitor the number of influenza-associated hospital and intensive care unit admissions. To allow for rapid data collection, NHSN, however, does not capture individual-level or in-depth clinical data on these hospitalizations.[3] By contrast, FluSurv-NET conducts population-based surveillance in 13 states that provides influenza hospitalization rates that can be stratified by demographic characteristics such as age or race/ethnicity. In addition, FluSurv-NET captures rich clinical data about persons hospitalized with influenza from multiple data sources, informing who is at increased risk for influenza-associated hospitalizations, the clinical characteristics and outcomes of influenza hospitalizations, and trends in influenza antiviral use and other treatment options. In addition, FluSurv-NET data can assess seasonal influenza severity and estimate influenza disease burden.[5,6] The complementary strengths of NHSN's real-time hospitalization data and FluSurv-NET's detailed clinical surveillance are integral parts of a national influenza surveillance system designed to inform

AJPH February 2026, Vol. 116, No. 2

timely interventions to prevent and control influenza.

PUBLIC HEALTH IMPLICATIONS

NHSN influenza hospitalization data are released weekly and geographically representative of the United States, making these data well-suited for nationwide influenza surveillance and forecasting. CDC's Influenza Division uses data from NHSN in its weekly surveillance summaries and current forecasting efforts.[1,7] Previous influenza forecasting efforts relied on outpatient surveillance for influenza-like illness and did not include all states and territories, and initial evaluations show these NHSN data have been useful for influenza forecasting.[8–10]

Beginning November 1, 2024, CMS implemented a new requirement for hospitals to electronically report information on COVID-19, influenza, and respiratory syncytial virus, in addition to bed capacity and occupancy, to NHSN to enhance situational awareness of respiratory disease.[11,12] Continuing to receive geographically representative, near-real-time influenza hospitalization data can inform seasonal influenza prevention and control efforts, pandemic preparedness, and health care system use and capacity. AJPH

ABOUT THE AUTHORS

Aaron M. Frutos, Shunte Moon, Catherine H. Bozio, Mark W. Tenforde, Matthew Biggerstaff, and Kelsey M. Sumner are with the Influenza Division, National Center for Immunization and Respiratory Diseases, Centers for Disease Control and Prevention (CDC), Atlanta, GA. Alison M. Binder and Margaret A. Dudeck are with the Division of Healthcare Quality Promotion, National Center for Emerging and Zoonotic Infectious Diseases, CDC. Andrea J. Cool, Kingsley Iyawe, and Trevor Thompson are with Booz Allen Hamilton, Atlanta.

CORRESPONDENCE

Correspondence should be sent to Kelsey M. Sumner, US Centers for Disease Control and Prevention, 1600 Clifton Rd, Atlanta, GA 30329 (e-mail: rhq3@cdc.gov). Reprints can be ordered at https://www.ajph.org by clicking the "Reprints" link.

PUBLICATION INFORMATION

Full Citation: Frutos AM, Moon S, Binder AM, et al. Evaluation of a novel data source for national influenza surveillance: influenza hospitalization data in the National Healthcare Safety Network, United States, September 2021–April 2024. *Am J Public Health*. 2026;116(2):251–255.

Acceptance Date: August 21, 2025.

DOI: https://doi.org/10.2105/AJPH.2025.308282

ORCID iDs:

Aaron M. Frutos https://orcid.org/0000-0001-6948-3918

Shunte Moon https://orcid.org/0000-0002-7243-7901

Alison M. Binder https://orcid.org/0000-0003-2726-3997

Trevor Thompson https://orcid.org/0009-0005-0226-395X

Margaret A. Dudeck https://orcid.org/0000-0001-8537-1940

Mark W. Tenforde https://orcid.org/0000-0002-8702-8393

Matthew Biggerstaff https://orcid.org/0000-0001-5108-8311

Kelsey M. Sumner https://orcid.org/0000-0002-4479-897X

CONTRIBUTORS

A. M. Frutos, S. Moon, M. W. Tenforde, M. Biggerstaff, and K. M. Sumner conceptualized the article. A. M. Frutos, A. J. Cool, K. Iyawe, and T. Thompson conducted statistical analyses and data management. A. M. Frutos, S. Moon, A. M. Binder, M. W. Tenforde, M. Biggerstaff, and K. M. Sumner provided methodology. S. Moon, A. M. Binder, M. A. Dudeck, and C. H. Bozio provided study investigation and coordination. S. Moon, M. W. Tenforde, M. Biggerstaff, and K. M. Sumner provided supervision. A. M. Frutos wrote the initial version of the article. All authors read and approved the final version of the article.

ACKNOWLEDGMENTS

The Influenza Hospitalization Surveillance Network (FluSurv-NET) is a collaboration of state health departments, academic institutions and local partners and is funded by the CDC. This work was supported by the CDC through an Emerging Infections Program cooperative agreement (grant CK17-1701) and through a Council of State and Territorial Epidemiologists cooperative agreement (grant NU38OT000297-02-00).

We thank all partners and participants.

Note. The findings and conclusions in this report are those of the authors and do not necessarily represent the views of the CDC. Some authors are federal employees of the US government, and this work was prepared as part of their official duties. Title 17 USC 105 provides that "copyright protection under this title is not available for any work of the United States Government."

CONFLICTS OF INTEREST

The authors have no conflicts of interest to report.

HUMAN PARTICIPANT PROTECTION

FluSurv-NET sites obtained human participants and ethics approval from their respective state health department, academic partner, and participating hospital institutional review boards as needed. This activity was reviewed by CDC, deemed not research, and was conducted consistent with applicable federal law and CDC policy (45 CFR part 46.102(l)(2); 21 CFR part 56; 42 USC Sect. 241(d); 5 USC Sect 552a; 44 USC Sect 3501 et seq.).

REFERENCES

1. Centers for Disease Control and Prevention. US influenza surveillance: purpose and methods. 2024. Available at: https://www.cdc.gov/fluview/overview. Accessed February 8, 2024.
2. Centers for Medicare and Medicaid Services. Updates to the Condition of Participation (CoP) Requirements for Hospitals and Critical Access Hospitals (CAHs) to Report Acute Respiratory Illnesses. Available at: https://www.cms.gov/medicare/health-safety-standards/quality-safety-oversight-general-information/policy-memos-states-and-cms-locations/updates-condition-participation-cop-requirements-hospitals-and-critical-access-hospitals-cahs-report. Accessed January 29, 2025.
3. National Healthcare Safety Network. Hospital respiratory data. Centers for Disease Control and Prevention. 2024. Available at: https://www.cdc.gov/nhsn/psc/hospital-respiratory-reporting.html. Accessed December 6, 2024.
4. Centers for Disease Control and Prevention. Influenza Hospitalization Surveillance Network (FluSurv-NET). 2023. Available at: https://www.cdc.gov/fluview/overview/influenza-hospitalization-surveillance.html. Accessed February 8, 2024,
5. Naquin A, O'Halloran A, Ujamaa D, et al. Laboratory-confirmed influenza-associated hospitalizations among children and adults—Influenza Hospitalization Surveillance Network, United States, 2010–2023. *MMWR Surveill Summ.* 2024;73(6):1–18. https://doi.org/10.15585/mmwr.ss7706a1
6. Centers for Disease Control and Prevention. How CDC classifies flu severity each season in the United States. 2024. Available at: https://www.cdc.gov/flu/php/surveillance. Accessed December 17, 2024.
7. Borchering RK, Biggerstaff M, Brammer L, et al. Responding to the return of influenza in the United States by applying Centers for Disease Control and Prevention surveillance, analysis, and modeling to inform understanding of seasonal influenza. *JMIR Public Health Surveill.* 2024;10:e54340. https://doi.org/10.2196/54340

8. Mathis SM, Webber AE, Leon TM, et al. Evaluation of FluSight influenza forecasting in the 2021–22 and 2022–23 seasons with a new target laboratory-confirmed influenza hospitalizations. Preprint. Posted online December 11, 2023. *medRxiv*. https://doi.org/10.1101/2023.12.08.23299726
9. Centers for Disease Control and Prevention. FluSight forecasting for influenza prevention and control. 2024. Available at: https://www.cdc.gov/flu-forecasting/about/index.html. Accessed March 1, 2024.
10. Couture A, Iuliano D, Chang HH, et al. State-level influenza hospitalization burden in the United States, 2022–2023. *Am J Public Health*. 2025;115(4):546–554. https://doi.org/10.2105/AJPH.2024.307928
11. Centers for Disease Control and Prevention. Updated hospital reporting requirements for respiratory viruses. 2024. Available at: https://www.cdc.gov/ncird/whats-new/updated-hospital-reporting-requirements-for-respiratory-viruses.html. Accessed December 6, 2024.
12. 2024 FY 2025 Hospital Inpatient Prospective Payment System (IPPS) and Long-Term Care Hospital Prospective Payment System (LTCH PPS) Final Rule—CMS-1808-F (US Centers for Medicare & Medicaid Services) 2462–2490. 2024. Available at: https://www.cms.gov/newsroom/fact-sheets/fy-2025-hospital-inpatient-prospective-payment-system-ipps-and-long-term-care-hospital-prospective-0. Accessed December 1, 2024.

Contextualizing President Trump's Executive Orders Targeting Transgender Health and Gender-Affirming Care

Nabiha Nuruzzaman, MD, MPH, and Elaine Hsiang, MD

See also xxxx.

The antitransgender executive orders and legislation enacted by the Trump administration since January 2025 have focused on enforcing a gender binary and restricting access to gender-affirming care for youths. These actions have had sweeping effects on health policy and access to care in an already strained health care system.

Here we contextualize these attacks on transgender health by exploring the historical pathologization and policing of transgender bodies in the United States and Europe while tracing the legacy of medical gatekeeping alongside evolving standards of care. We critique the scientific inaccuracies within the administration's executive orders while outlining the harmful impact of related and recent legislation, including *United States v Skrmetti*.

Restrictions on gender-affirming care and the rights of transgender people to exist not only exacerbate health disparities but also undermine the ethical responsibility of medical practitioners and institutions to provide patient-centered, evidence-based care. We must not capitulate to political efforts that attempt to harm and erase an already marginalized population. (*Am J Public Health*. 2026;116(2):256–260. https://doi.org/10.2105/AJPH.2025.308265)

AJPH February 2026, Vol. 116, No. 2

Building on the promises of a virulently antitransgender campaign, US President Donald Trump released several executive orders shortly after taking office, including Defending Women from Gender Ideology Extremism and Restoring Biological Truth to the Federal Government[1] (January 20, 2025) and Protecting Children from Chemical and Surgical Mutilation[2] (January 28, 2025). According to the former executive order,

> It is the policy of the United States to recognize two sexes, male and female. These sexes are not changeable and are grounded in fundamental and incontrovertible reality.[1]

The latter declares,

> It is the policy of the United States that it will not fund, sponsor, promote, assist or support the so-called "transition" of a child from one sex to another and it will rigorously enforce all laws that prohibit or limit these destructive and life-altering procedures.[2]

These orders and subsequent presidential declarations contain assertions that are scientifically inaccurate and represent a massive overreach by federal authority to intimidate health care institutions to comply with oppressive ideologies that purport the false claim that gender-affirming care for youths constitutes child abuse. Furthermore, by defining a "child" as anyone younger than 19 years, the executive order deliberately blurs the line between minors and adults to justify future broader restrictions on adult health care.[2]

In the weeks after these orders, multiple hospital systems—including in California, Colorado, New York, Virginia, and Washington—preemptively halted gender-affirming appointments and procedures for patients younger than 19 years, compromising patients reliant on this care.[3] Protests sprung up as thousands of patients, families, and allies advocated for the resumption of gender-affirming care at these institutions and contested the legality of the current administration's actions.[3] Federal lawsuits and temporary restraining orders have since been filed against both of these executive orders,[3] but the long-term effects on health care access, nondiscrimination protections, and federal funding remain uncertain.

LEGACY OF BINARY GENDER NORMS

Although these efforts to enforce gender as a binary reflect a renewed partisan intensity, they are not without precedent. The historical policing of transgender bodies in America is a complex narrative tied to normative constructions of sex, race, and gender and shaped by societal attempts to pathologize gender diversity. The targeting of transgender people is deeply rooted in patriarchal gender norms imposed by Western Christian societies, exemplified by the destruction of Magnus Hirschfeld's work in Germany.

Magnus Hirschfeld founded the Institute for Sexual Research in 1919 in Berlin, establishing a groundbreaking center for medical, anthropological, and psychological inquiry into the growing field of sexology.[4] The institute was notable for its pioneering work and treatment of people whose bodies did not match their assigned genders at birth but also offered various modes of social support, including employment and political advocacy, for its clients.[4] Hirschfeld introduced the term "sexual intermediaries" for nonconforming individuals, which included "transvestites," a term he coined in 1910 to describe a "much wider range of transsexual and transgender phenomena and identities."[4]

The institute's association with both homosexuality and Jewishness made it an early target of Nazi violence. In 1933, the institute was raided, with a large part of its collection subjected to book burning.[4] Hirschfeld's work, in recognizing the plurality of gender identity and sexual behavior, faced violent repression, which shifted the center of sexological inquiry to the United States. This serves as a stark warning for the present moment as we confront state-sanctioned efforts that attempt to erase transgender existence.

In contemporary society, transgender individuals continue to be positioned as threats disrupting the legitimacy of binary and fixed gender. Their bodies remain "hotly contested site[s] of cultural inscription"[5(p164)] subject to unprecedented levels of violence. The executive orders coincide with a series of federal initiatives that target transgender visibility and existence, including in the military, college sports, and the national workforce, often disproportionately targeting transgender women through "transphobic spatial segregation."[6] The targeted focus on transgender youths in these policies reveals attempts to engineer a future based on a binary gender fantasy, echoing historical eugenic ideologies. Youths, as a legally and socially vulnerable group, have limited power to contest attacks on their rights. Legal scholar Naomi Cahn describes how the rhetoric of parental rights is wielded "as a Trojan horse for. . .banning gender-affirming care. . .regardless of what parents actually want,"[7] often serving as a smokescreen for harmful policies over evidence-based interventions that actually support youths.

GATEKEEPING CARE VIA PATHOLOGIZATION AND MEDICALIZATION

Endocrinologist and sexologist Harry Benjamin is often credited with defining transsexuality as a desire to change sex.[8] Benjamin worked with other sexologists, including Hirschfeld, across Europe and the United States and argued that transsexuality could be treated through medical and surgical interventions. The term "transgender" later emerged "as an attempt to forge a politics and sense of community around the demedicalized desire to be differently gendered."[9(p111)]

Although pioneering what would become gender-affirming care, Benjamin's framework was deeply problematic and influenced by the eugenic ideology pervasive throughout the United States in the 19th and early 20th centuries. Benjamin practiced extensive medical gatekeeping, defined as enforcing strict psychological and behavioral criteria patients had to meet to be determined as fit to access transition-related services.[8,10]

An archival investigation of Benjamin's clinic documents by medical sociologist stef shuster highlights the ways in which eugenics determined who was considered an ideal patient.[10] "Old" eugenics exerted reproductive control over transgender people by encouraging them to leave their families and children after transitioning. "New" eugenics focused on maintaining social order and social control over transgender patients by selecting the ideal patients to undergo transition. Patients had to conform to traditional gender norms and be perceived as able to "pass" as their identified gender after transitioning; transgender women who were too masculine or transgender men who were too feminine were dismissed as social failures undeserving of medical transition.

To reduce legal risks, Benjamin required patients to undergo a mental health assessment to screen out those who were mentally unstable or challenged medical authority. This practice reflected the deliberate pathologization of transgender identity. shuster describes who was left to access gender-affirming care:

> Transgender people who were compliant to authority, white, middle-class, gainfully employed and desired to be in heterosexual relationships upon transitioning were held in the highest regard as 'ideal' patients.[10(p209)]

These narrow criteria meant the denial of medical care for many and reinforced the idea that only certain bodies were worthy of health care. This was reflected in low rates of acceptance into the gender identity clinics at major research universities in the 1960s and 1970s.[8] Established in 1968, the Stanford Gender Dysphoria Program was one of the first clinics in the United States to provide care to transgender people. Academic theorist Sandy Stone described the highly selective, yet arbitrary, process by which medical providers at that clinic determined treatment eligibility on the basis of subjective views of patients' performance in their identified gender and whether their sexual expression was socially acceptable.[5] These criteria not only forced gender conformity but also conflated sexual and gender identity during a time in which transsexuality was still commonly considered indistinct from homosexuality.

In 1979, the Harry Benjamin International Gender Dysphoria Association, which would later become the World Professional Association for Transgender Health (WPATH), released its first Standards of Care guidelines for gender-affirming care.[8] The initial guidelines were written by cisgender authors and relied heavily on Benjamin's gatekeeping model, mandating mental health assessments, psychotherapy, and a period of social transition before patients could access gender-affirming therapies.[11] In 1980, the third edition of the *Diagnostic and Statistical Manual of Mental Disorders* (*DSM*) introduced "gender identity disorder" as a formal psychiatric diagnosis in which transgender identity was pathologized within a binary and medicalized narrative.[11] Access to care was deliberately restricted, forcing transgender patients to strategically engage with a cisheteronormative system that labeled them as having a mental disorder.

It was not until the 1990s that transgender voices were included in Standards of Care revisions. Criticism and advocacy by transgender communities and their allies have contributed to key changes in subsequent versions of the guidelines. For example, Kenneth Zucker, a psychologist and sexologist who recommended the dangerous model of conversion therapy, was a coauthor until he was deplatformed from WPATH in 2017.[8] In 2013, the fifth edition of the *DSM* replaced gender identity disorder with gender dysphoria, describing instead the distress experienced as a result of gender incongruence and marking the gradual transition to more affirming care models and informed consent.[11]

Because of continued criticisms that WPATH guidelines can be exclusionary and paternalistic, the current standards (Standards of Care 8), released in 2022, have begun to shift toward a model of shared decision making. These and other changes reflect ongoing conversations between transgender health experts, patients, and advocates to design guidelines and best practices that are meant to serve and validate the transgender community in a health care system that has historically restricted its members' access to care.

Despite progress made in transgender health, acceptance of gender-affirming care is often hindered by discourses popularized by legislators that fixate on discussions of "transgender regret" or "detransition" as a phenomenon. In addition, the ongoing contestation of whether gender-affirming care is considered "medically necessary" by insurance providers reinforces gatekeeping tactics by health care systems and political authorities.[11] Transgender scholars have written about the need to depathologize transness and make gender-affirming care available as a human right without subscribing to a narrative that conditions medical care on the premise of curing gender dysphoria.[8]

CURRENT DISPARITIES IN TRANSGENDER HEALTH

Transgender health disparities are well documented in the literature. Transgender people experience disproportionately worse medical and mental health outcomes than cisgender populations, in large part because of compounded discrimination, stigma, and denial of care in health care settings.[12,13] Recent research suggests that transgender health inequities have worsened over the past decade, alongside the dramatic rise in antitransgender legislation and the denial of not only basic human rights but also access to comprehensive and compassionate health care, including gender-affirming care.[13,14]

Gender-affirming care remains a hotly politicized topic, yet gender-affirming therapies are most often used for cisgender people[15,16]; common indications include hormone replacement therapy for menopause, precocious pubertal suppression, reconstructive mammoplasty after mastectomy, depilation for unwanted hair growth, and fertility preservation before cancer treatment. Among transgender youths, gender-affirming medical and surgical therapies have been found to reduce gender dysphoria, mood disorders, and suicidality,[17,18] with widespread acknowledgment by leading medical societies[19] that gender-affirming care is life saving and medically necessary. The notion that treatments used to help cisgender people live as their authentic selves are pathologized for transgender people raises the question of who, then, is allowed to access gender-affirming care? It is clear that discriminatory policies will be applied to those whom the antitransgender populace does not believe should exist. The recognition of gender-affirming care as a right, rather than a medical exception, is a critical step to providing equitable health care for those of all gender identities.

IMPACT OF GENDER-AFFIRMING HEALTH CARE BANS

The executive order titled Protecting Children from Chemical and Surgical Mutilation criticizes WPATH for lacking scientific integrity and demands that institutions rescind reliance on the organization's guidelines.[2] However, the order fails to provide credible evidence to support this claim. At the direction of President Trump, the Department of Health and Human Services published a literature review in May 2025 claiming that gender-affirming care is harmful. [20] This report, whose authors are undisclosed, is widely viewed as part of a broader anti-transgender agenda and has drawn sharp criticism for contradicting scientific evidence, promoting misinformation, and endorsing discredited concepts such as "rapid onset gender dysphoria" while encouraging conversion therapy.[20]

The surge of antitransgender legislation, fueled by antiabortion Christian and conservative groups challenging established medical consensus, contributes to the systematic discrimination, social isolation, and interpersonal violence that transgender people regularly navigate in daily American life.[21] These initiatives, including Arkansas's ban on gender-affirming care for minors and Texas's executive injunction that gender-affirming care should be prosecuted as child abuse, falsely portray transgender youths as needing protection from "criminal" health care providers or their supportive parents and guardians.[22] Although there is substantial evidence linking the detrimental mental health impact of these discriminatory laws, this evidence continues to be ignored.[14] In Utah, lawmakers upholding the state's moratorium on gender-affirming care for minors dismissed a state-commissioned report published in May 2025 that demonstrated that gender-affirming care is associated with improved mental health and psychosocial outcomes.[23]

In June 2025, the US Supreme Court upheld Tennessee's ban on gender-affirming care for minors in *United States v Skrmetti*, determining that the law does not constitute sex-based discrimination or violate the Equal Protection Clause of the 14th Amendment.[22] This decision not only preserves similar bans in 25 states but also sets a precedent that may enable future state efforts to restrict care for adults. Alongside *United States v Skrmetti*, the current administration's executive orders affect safe haven states that offer legal protections for patients traveling to receive gender-affirming care.[3] Across the United States, the growing number of restrictions on transgender health has already limited access to care based on race, geographic location, and socioeconomic status.[22]

Gender-affirming care typically involves highly individualized treatments developed through multidisciplinary collaborations and evidence-based protocols. In practice, patients often wrestle with long wait times, extensive travel, insurance-related issues, and medical gatekeeping. Additional bans on gender-affirming care are likely to increase risks to both patients and their health care providers. As state-level variation in transgender legislation is known to affect individual health care access,[24] executive orders and legislative actions targeting medical access among transgender youths are poised to widen national health care disparities in an already strained and complex health care system.

ROLE OF THE MEDICAL ESTABLISHMENT

The reactionary suspension of gender-affirming care by private institutions has immediate and significant public health consequences. Limiting access to gender-affirming care for transgender individuals increases health disparities, worsens health outcomes, and erodes trust in the health care system. Health care institutions have a responsibility to uphold established, evidence-based standards and should avoid proactive compliance with harmful policies that sign off on the discriminatory tactics of this administration. Institutions must also support their providers and stand against efforts to restrict scientific funding or interfere with the patient–provider relationship. Above all, it is our ethical obligation as health care professionals to safeguard and expand access to gender-affirming care while confronting the oppressive ideologies that threaten the health and rights of transgender people. AJPH

ABOUT THE AUTHORS

The authors are with the Department of Emergency Medicine, Stanford University School of Medicine, Palo Alto, CA.

CORRESPONDENCE

Correspondence should be sent to Nabiha Nuruzzaman, MD, MPH, Department of Emergency Medicine, Stanford University School of Medicine, 900 Welch Rd, Suite 350, Palo Alto, CA 94304 (e-mail: nabiha@stanford.edu). Reprints can be ordered at https://www.ajph.org by clicking the "Reprints" link.

PUBLICATION INFORMATION

Full Citation: Nuruzzaman N, Hsiang E. Contextualizing President Trump's executive orders targeting transgender health and gender-affirming care. *Am J Public Health*. 2026;116(2):256–260.

Acceptance Date: August 1, 2025.

DOI: https://doi.org/10.2105/AJPH.2025.308265

ORCID iDs:
Nabiha Nuruzzaman https://orcid.org/0000-0001-9921-2991

Elaine Hsiang https://orcid.org/0000-0002-1393-8204

CONTRIBUTORS

The authors contributed equally to this work.

CONFLICTS OF INTEREST

The authors have no conflicts of interest.

HUMAN PARTICIPANT PROTECTION

No human participants were involved.

REFERENCES

1. The White House. Defending women from gender ideology extremism and restoring biological truth to the federal government. Available at: https://www.whitehouse.gov/presidential-actions/2025/01/defending-women-from-gender-ideology-extremism-and-restoring-biological-truth-to-the-federal-government. Accessed April 5, 2025.
2. The White House. Protecting children from chemical and surgical mutilation. Available at: https://www.whitehouse.gov/presidential-actions/2025/01/protecting-children-from-chemical-and-surgical-mutilation. Accessed April 5, 2025.
3. KFF. Overview of President Trump's executive actions impacting LGBTQ+ health. Available at: https://www.kff.org/other/fact-sheet/overview-of-president-trumps-executive-actions-impacting-lgbtq-health. Accessed April 5, 2025.
4. Bauer H, Blume S, Greenough P. From fragile solidarities to burnt sexual subjects: at the Institute of Sexual Science. Available at: https://www.jstor.org/stable/j.ctt1wf4dmd.8?seq=3. Accessed April 5, 2025.
5. Stone S. The empire strikes back: a posttranssexual manifesto. *Camera Obscura*. 1992;10(2):150–176. https://doi.org/10.1215/02705346-10-2_29-150
6. Bagagli BP, Chaves TV, Fontana MGZ. Trans women and public restrooms: the legal discourse and its violence. *Front Sociol*. 2021;6:652777. Published online https://doi.org/10.3389/fsoc.2021.652777
7. Cahn N. The political language of parental rights: abortion, gender-affirming care, and critical race theory. Available at: https://scholarship.shu.edu/cgi/viewcontent.cgi?article=3549&context=shlr. Accessed April 5, 2025.
8. Amin K. Trans negative affect. Available at: https://static1.squarespace.com/static/61f079015ffca22cceca0594/t/63b4ad3146d97c152a94ea95/1672785201308/AminTransNegativeAffect.pdf. Accessed April 5, 2025.
9. Amin K. We are all nonbinary: a brief history of accidents. *Representations*. 2022;158(1):106–119. https://doi.org/10.1525/rep.2022.158.11.106
10. shuster s. The assertion of reproductive and social control in mid-twentieth-century US transgender medicine. *Gender History*. 2024;36(1):208–223. https://doi.org/10.1111/1468-0424.12727
11. Dietz E. More necessary than medical: reframing the insurance argument for transition-related care. *Int J Feminist Approaches Bioethics*. 2020;13(1):63–88. https://doi.org/10.3138/ijfab.13.1.04
12. Streed CG, McCarthy EP, Haas JS. Association between gender minority status and self-reported physical and mental health in the United States. *JAMA Intern Med*. 2017;177(8):1210–1212. https://doi.org/10.1001/jamainternmed.2017.1460
13. Restar AJ, Layland EK, Davis B, Thompson H, Streed C. The public health crisis state of transgender health care and policy. *Am J Public Health*. 2024;114(2):161–163. https://doi.org/10.2105/ajph.2023.307523
14. Liu M, Patel VR, Reisner SL, Keuroghlian AS. Health status and mental health of transgender and gender-diverse adults. *JAMA Intern Med*. 2024;184(8):984–986. https://doi.org/10.1001/jamainternmed.2024.2544
15. Schall TE, Moses JD. Gender-affirming care for cisgender people. *Hastings Cent Rep*. 2023;53(3):15–24. https://doi.org/10.1002/hast.1486
16. Budge SL, Abreu RL, Flinn RE, et al. Gender affirming care is evidence based for transgender and gender-diverse youth. *J Adolesc Health*. 2024;75(6):851–853. https://doi.org/10.1016/j.jadohealth.2024.09.009
17. Olson-Kennedy J, Warus J, Okonta V, Belzer M, Clark LF. Chest reconstruction and chest dysphoria in transmasculine minors and young adults. *JAMA Pediatr*. 2018;172(5):431–436. https://doi.org/10.1001/jamapediatrics.2017.5440
18. Tordoff DM, Wanta JW, Collin A, Stepney C, Inwards-Breland DJ, Ahrens K. Mental health outcomes in transgender and nonbinary youths receiving gender-affirming care. *JAMA Netw Open*. 2022;5(2):e220978. https://doi.org/10.1001/jamanetworkopen.2022.0978
19. GLAAD. Medical association statements in support of health care for transgender people and youth. Available at: https://glaad.org/medical-association-statements-supporting-trans-youth-healthcare-and-against-discriminatory. Accessed April 5, 2025.
20. Kates J, Dawson L, Park M, Musumeci MUS. Department of Health and Human Services report on pediatric gender dysphoria and gender conversion efforts. Available at: https://www.kff.org/mental-health/issue-brief/u-s-department-of-health-and-human-services-report-on-pediatric-gender-dysphoria-and-gender-conversion-efforts. Accessed April 5, 2025.
21. Contreras R. The forces behind anti-trans bills across the US. Available at: https://www.axios.com/2023/03/31/anti-trans-bills-2023-america. Accessed April 5, 2025.
22. Dawson L, Kates J. Gender-affirming care policy tracker. Available at: https://www.kff.org/other/dashboard/gender-affirming-care-policy-tracker. Accessed April 5, 2025.
23. Utah Department of Health and Human Services. Systematic medical evidence review of hormonal transgender treatment report. Available at: https://le.utah.gov/AgencyRP/reportingDetail.jsp?rid=636. Accessed April 5, 2025.
24. Tran NK, Baker KE, Lett E, Scheim AI. State-level heterogeneity in associations between structural stigma and individual health care access: a multilevel analysis of transgender adults in the United States. *J Health Serv Res Policy*. 2023;28(2):109–118. https://doi.org/10.1177/13558196221123413

Association of Discrimination and Violence With Suicidality Among *Travestis* and Transgender Women in Rio de Janeiro, Brazil, 2015–2023: A Cross-Sectional Study

David R. A. Coelho, MD, MPH, Emilia M. Jalil, MD, PhD, Biancka Fernandes, Eduardo Peixoto, PhD, Thaylla Vianna, Michele Ramos, MD, Cristina M. Jalil, PhD, Livia Ferreira, MD, Isabele Barboza Moura, MSc, Ruth K. Friedman, MD, PhD, Arthur Chaves Araujo, MA, Sandra Cardoso Wagner, MD, PhD, Sari L. Reisner, ScD, Alex S. Keuroghlian, MD, MPH, Valdiléa G. Veloso, MD, PhD, Beatriz Grinsztejn, MD, PhD, and Carolina Coutinho, PhD

See also Scheim, p. 166.

AJPH February 2026, Vol. 116, No. 2

Objectives. To examine the associations between discrimination, violence, and suicidality among *travestis* and transgender women in Brazil.

Methods. We analyzed baseline data from the *Transcendendo* cohort (2015–2023) in Rio de Janeiro, Brazil, which enrolled *travestis* and transgender women aged 18 years and older. We assessed lifetime discrimination by using an 8-item scale reflecting transgender-related mistreatment experiences. We also measured physical and sexual violence, sociodemographics, and psychosocial factors. We categorized suicidality as no ideation, ideation only, and ideation with attempts, analyzed using a multivariable ordinal regression model.

Results. Among 662 participants, lifetime discrimination (adjusted odds ratio [AOR] = 1.21; 95% confidence interval [CI] = 1.11, 1.32; $P < .001$) and lifetime sexual assault (AOR = 1.60; 95% CI = 1.17, 2.19; $P = .003$) were significantly associated with increased odds of suicidality. Participants with positive body self-satisfaction, HIV, and increasing age had lower odds of suicidality.

Conclusions. Our findings highlight the need for antidiscriminatory policies and health services tailored to the needs of this community to mitigate suicidality risk among *travestis* and transgender women in Brazil. (*Am J Public Health*. 2026;116(2):261–269. https://doi.org/10.2105/AJPH.2025.308280)

Travestis and transgender women (TGW) in Brazil face social and health disparities exacerbated by discrimination and violence,[1] with the country recording a high number of murders of transgender, nonbinary, and gender-diverse people, with TGW being the most affected.[2] This pervasive context of transphobia, characterized by policies, practices, and norms that systematically discriminate, marginalize, and oppress transgender, nonbinary, and gender-diverse people, leads not only to restricted access to education and employment but also to significant health disparities.[3] This includes a disproportionate burden of HIV and mental health conditions within this marginalized community.[1,4]

Suicidality, encompassing both suicidal ideation and attempts, is a public health concern. According to the World Health Organization, suicide accounts for 700 000 deaths worldwide each year.[5] A meta-analysis found that 50% of transgender, nonbinary, and gender-diverse people experienced suicidal thoughts, and 29% had attempted suicide over their lifetime.[6] Research has demonstrated that discrimination and violence are associated with suicidality among different populations.[1,7] Discrimination in various forms (e.g., job, academic, health care, or social settings) precipitates trauma and chronic stress.[8] These conditions may contribute to suicidal ideation and attempts, which, in Brazil, may be further exacerbated by endemic violence against transgender and gender-diverse communities.[2]

Previous studies in Rio de Janeiro, Brazil, have associated discrimination and violence with mental health outcomes among TGW.[1,9] One study identified associations with depressive symptoms,[1] while another examined suicidal ideation and suicide attempts.[9] However, less is known about how these factors correlate with suicidality as an ordinal variable. Ideation-to-action theories of suicidality posit a progression from suicidal ideation to suicide attempts and underscore the importance of understanding the distinct mechanisms underlying these processes.[10] This study aimed to address this gap by assessing the associations of discrimination, physical violence, and sexual violence with suicidality among TGW, using an ordinal measure to capture varying levels of suicidal behavior.

METHODS

This was a cross-sectional study analyzing baseline survey data from the *Transcendendo* cohort, from August 2015 (cohort establishment) to December 2023, conducted in Rio de Janeiro.

Study Population

Inclusion criteria consisted of participants aged 18 years and older; assigned male sex at birth; identifying as *travestis* (a gender identity within the transfeminine spectrum that is culturally specific to Latin America, particularly Brazil),[11] transgender women, women, or another gender along the transfeminine spectrum; and living in Rio de Janeiro or its metropolitan regions. Exclusion criteria included any condition that could impair the ability to provide informed consent or accurately respond to the questionnaire, such as substance intoxication. Participants were enrolled via 3 key pathways: (1) referrals from *Transcender*, a respondent-driven sampling–based study conducted at our institution with subsequent open-door enrollment; (2) TGW who actively sought participation in research or accessed health related services at the study site; and (3) those already enrolled in an HIV clinical cohort. Data were collected through comprehensive interviews conducted in person by trained professionals in a space reserved for this purpose. In cases of any identified mental health condition, participants were systematically directed to mental health services within our center or designated health centers within the Brazilian Public Health System (*Sistema Único de Saúde* [SUS]), which provides health care free of charge for all people.

Variables Analyzed

Sociodemographic, psychosocial, and HIV status characteristics. Sociodemographic variables were age (continuous), race/ethnicity (Black/*Parda*, White, and other), educational level (8 years of education representing the threshold for secondary education completion in Brazil), daily income (US $1.90 serving as the benchmark for extreme poverty as defined by the World Bank in 2015 at the establishment of the cohort), and relationship status (single vs having a partner). *Parda* refers to a mixed-race identity commonly used in Brazilian demographic classifications.[12] We recategorized sexual orientation into heterosexual, homosexual, and other (bisexual, asexual, and pansexual), given the predominant representation of heterosexual orientation within this cohort of TGW and the low frequency of other sexual orientations to calculate estimates for them. Other relevant variables included self-reported HIV status and psychosocial factors such as current gender-affirming hormone therapy, body self-satisfaction, and self-rated health quality. We analyzed each as a binary variable.

Exposures of interest. One of our exposures of interest was lifetime discrimination, assessed through a specific interview question. We quantified discrimination using a scale consisting of 8 items designed to capture various aspects of lifetime discriminatory experiences attributable to the transgender, nonbinary, and gender-diverse identities of participants. The items encompassed scenarios that included difficulties in securing employment, job termination, eviction from housing or educational institutions, challenges in accessing health care services, verbal abuse, and discrimination from friends or family. Participants responded to each item with "yes" or "no." A cumulative discrimination score was derived by totaling the affirmative responses, with possible scores ranging from 0 to 8. Higher scores indicated a greater extent of experienced discrimination throughout the participant's lifetime. Our 2 other exposures of interest were lifetime physical and sexual violence. We evaluated physical violence with the binary question: "Have you ever been physically hurt because of your trans identity?" Similarly, we assessed sexual assault with the binary question: "Have you ever been forced to have sexual intercourse against your will?" Responses to these questions were recorded as either "yes" or "no."

Outcome of interest. Our outcome of interest was suicidality. Applying an ideation-to-action suicidality framework, which emphasizes the importance of analyzing suicidality as a progression from ideation to attempts,[10] we categorized suicidality into 3 ordinal levels for this analysis: (1) no suicidal ideation and no suicide attempt, (2) suicidal ideation but no suicide attempt, and (3) suicidal ideation and suicide attempt. To assess this, we used specific interview questions from participant assessments in our center: suicidal ideation was determined by asking, "Have you ever thought about killing yourself?" and suicide attempts were assessed with the question, "Have you ever tried to kill yourself?" Responses to these questions were recorded as either "yes" or "no."

Statistical Analysis

Variables are descriptively presented with medians and interquartile ranges (IQRs) for continuous variables, and total counts along with percentages for categorical variables. Both bivariable and multivariable analyses utilized ordinal regression to estimate the odds ratios (ORs) and 95% confidence intervals (CIs) for suicidality.

The ordinal regression model was well-suited for this analysis because it allowed the examination of suicidality as a hierarchy of severity. Specifically, it modeled the ordinal nature of the outcomes (1) no suicidal ideation and no suicide attempt, (2) suicidal ideation but no suicide attempt, and (3) suicidal ideation and suicide attempt. By doing so, the model provided insights into the odds of falling into a higher category of suicidality versus a lower one, capturing the progression of suicidal behaviors.

We conducted variable selection for the multivariable model using a backward stepwise method, retaining predictors with a significance level of $P \le .20$ (body self-satisfaction and self-rated health quality), as recommended for stepwise modeling.[13] We also adjusted the model for sociodemographic and HIV-related variables, such as age, race/ethnicity, education, daily income, and HIV status. Our final multivariable model included our 3 exposures of interest, the sociodemographic variables and HIV status, and the 2 variables selected by the stepwise method. Before conducting the regression analyses, we verified and met the assumptions of proportional odds. In addition, we assessed multicollinearity, and none of the selected variables had a variance inflation factor greater than 5. We performed statistical analysis using R version 4.0.2 (R Foundation for Statistical Computing, Vienna, Austria), and we considered $P \le .05$ statistically significant.

RESULTS

A total of 938 TGW were enrolled in the cohort between 2015 and 2023. Of these, 22 had missing data for our outcome and 254 had missing data for other variables. Given the absence of any discernible pattern in the missing data, we conducted a complete-case analysis. Consequently, the current analysis included data from 662 TGW.

Overall, the median age was 31 years (IQR = 25–39), with 73.7% identifying as Black/*Parda*, 66.8% having more than 8 years of education, 15.9% earning less than US $1.90 per day, 70.7% being heterosexual, and 82.3% being single (Table 1). Most TGW surveyed were not on gender-affirming hormone therapy (52.9%) and self-reported positive body satisfaction and positive health quality (89.1% and 62.7%, respectively). A majority of the sample self-reported living with HIV (53.2%), and 66.8% reported ever engagement in sex work. The median lifetime discrimination score was 4 (IQR = 2–5); 53.3% had a history of physical violence and 44.3% of sexual assault. A total of 51.5% screened positive for lifetime suicidal ideation or suicide attempts (23.4% suicidal ideation only, and 28.1% suicidal ideation and suicide attempts). The annual distribution of suicidality from 2015 to 2023 is presented in Table A (available as a supplement to the online version of this article at https://ajph.org).

The bivariable analysis demonstrated significant associations of discrimination and violence with suicidality. Each unit increase in lifetime discrimination score was associated with higher odds of suicidality (OR = 1.30; 95% CI = 1.20, 1.40; $P < .001$). Lifetime physical violence (OR = 1.87; 95% CI = 1.40, 2.50; $P < .001$) and sexual assault (OR = 1.96; 95% CI = 1.46, 2.62; $P < .001$) were also associated with higher odds of suicidality (Table 2).

In the multivariable analysis (full model shown in Table 2), each unit increase in lifetime discrimination score (adjusted odds ratio [AOR] = 1.21; 95% CI = 1.11, 1.32; $P < .001$) and lifetime sexual assault (AOR = 1.60; 95% CI = 1.17, 2.19; $P = .003$) remained significantly associated with higher odds of suicidality. Lifetime physical violence was not statistically significant in the multivariable analysis (AOR = 1.28; 95% CI = 0.91, 1.79; $P = .15$). Positive body self-satisfaction (AOR = 0.48; 95% CI = 0.30, 0.77; $P = .002$) was associated with lower odds of suicidality, whereas positive self-rated health quality (AOR = 0.73; 95% CI = 0.53, 1.00; $P = .053$) was not. Participants who self-reported living with HIV had lower odds of suicidality

TABLE 1— Characteristics of the Study Population Overall and According to Suicidality Among *Travestis* and Transgender Women Enrolled in the *Transcendendo* Cohort: Rio de Janeiro, Brazil, 2015–2023

Variable	Descriptive Analysis, Median (IQR) or No. (%)			
	Overall, n = 662 (100%)	No Suicidal Ideation and No Suicide Attempt, n = 321 (48.5%)	Suicidal Ideation and No Suicide Attempt, n = 155 (23.4%)	Suicidal Ideation and Suicide Attempt, n = 186 (28.1%)
Age, y	31 (25–39)	32 (25–40)	31 (25–39)	29 (24–36)
Race/ethnicity				
Black/*Parda*	488 (73.7)	245 (76.3)	105 (67.7)	138 (74.2)
Other	11 (1.7)	3 (0.9)	4 (2.6)	4 (2.1)
White	163 (24.6)	73 (22.8)	46 (29.7)	44 (23.7)
Education, y				
≤ 8	220 (33.2)	118 (36.8)	46 (29.7)	56 (30.1)
> 8	442 (66.8)	203 (63.2)	109 (70.3)	130 (69.9)
Daily income,[a] US $				
≤ 1.90	105 (15.9)	44 (13.7)	26 (16.8)	35 (18.8)
> 1.90	557 (84.1)	277 (86.3)	129 (83.2)	151 (81.2)
Sexual orientation				
Heterosexual	468 (70.7)	222 (69.2)	117 (75.5)	129 (69.4)
Homosexual	111 (16.8)	65 (20.3)	19 (12.3)	27 (14.5)
Other	35 (5.3)	12 (3.7)	7 (4.5)	16 (8.6)
Relationship status				
Single	545 (82.3)	268 (83.5)	129 (83.2)	148 (79.6)
Having a partner	117 (17.7)	53 (16.5)	26 (16.8)	38 (20.4)
Current GAHT				
No	350 (52.9)	174 (54.2)	86 (55.5)	90 (48.4)
Yes	312 (47.1)	147 (45.8)	69 (44.5)	96 (51.6)
Body self-satisfaction				
Negative	72 (10.9)	19 (5.9)	21 (13.5)	32 (17.2)
Positive	590 (89.1)	302 (94.1)	134 (86.5)	154 (82.8)
Self-rated health quality				
Negative	247 (37.3)	100 (31.2)	64 (41.3)	83 (44.6)
Positive	415 (62.7)	221 (68.8)	91 (58.7)	103 (55.4)
Self-reported HIV status				
Not with HIV	310 (46.8)	134 (41.7)	74 (47.7)	102 (54.8)
With HIV	352 (53.2)	187 (58.3)	81 (52.3)	84 (45.2)
Lifetime sex work				
No	220 (33.2)	102 (31.8)	51 (32.9)	67 (36)
Yes	442 (66.8)	219 (68.2)	104 (67.1)	119 (64)
Lifetime discrimination score	4 (2–5)	3 (2–5)	4 (3–5)	5 (3–6)
Lifetime physical violence				
No	309 (46.7)	173 (53.9)	73 (47.1)	63 (33.9)
Yes	353 (53.3)	148 (46.1)	82 (52.9)	123 (66.1)
Lifetime sexual assault				
No	369 (55.7)	205 (63.9)	84 (54.2)	80 (43)
Yes	293 (44.3)	116 (36.1)	71 (45.8)	106 (57)

Note. GAHT = gender-affirming hormone therapy; IQR = interquartile range.
[a]US $1.90 served as the benchmark for extreme poverty, as defined by the World Bank in 2015 at the establishment of the cohort.

TABLE 2— Analysis of Suicidality Among *Travestis* and Transgender Women Enrolled in the *Transcendendo* Cohort: Rio de Janeiro, Brazil, 2015–2023

Variable	Bivariable Model, OR (95% CI)	Multivariable Model, AOR (95% CI)
Age	0.98 (0.96, 0.99)	0.98 (0.97, 1.00)
Race/ethnicity		
Black/*Parda*	0.89 (0.64, 1.24)	0.90 (0.63, 1.27)
Other	1.73 (0.58, 5.25)	1.54 (0.51, 4.74)
White (Ref)	1	1
Education		
≤ 8 y (Ref)	1	1
> 8 y	1.31 (0.96, 1.79)	1.33 (0.96, 1.85)
Daily income,[a] US $		
≤ 1.90 (Ref)	1	1
> 1.90	0.74 (0.50, 1.08)	0.94 (0.62, 1.41)
Sexual orientation		
Heterosexual (Ref)	1	...
Homosexual	0.70 (0.46, 1.04)	...
Other	1.38 (0.89, 2.13)	...
Relationship status		
Single (Ref)	1	...
Having a partner	1.22 (0.84, 1.77)	...
Current GAHT		
No (Ref)	1	...
Yes	1.17 (0.88, 1.56)	...
Body self-satisfaction		
Negative (Ref)	1	1
Positive	0.40 (0.25, 0.63)	0.48 (0.30, 0.77)
Self-rated health quality		
Negative (Ref)	1	1
Positive	0.62 (0.46, 0.83)	0.73 (0.53, 1.00)
Self-reported HIV status		
Not with HIV (Ref)	1	1
With HIV	0.66 (0.49, 0.88)	0.68 (0.50, 0.92)
Lifetime sex work		
No (Ref)	1	...
Yes	0.87 (0.64, 1.17)	...
Lifetime discrimination score	1.30 (1.20, 1.40)	1.21 (1.11, 1.32)
Lifetime physical violence		
No (Ref)	1	1
Yes	1.87 (1.40, 2.50)	1.28 (0.91, 1.79)
Lifetime sexual assault		
No (Ref)	1	1
Yes	1.96 (1.46, 2.62)	1.60 (1.17, 2.19)

Note. AOR = adjusted odds ratio; CI = confidence interval; GAHT = gender-affirming hormone therapy; OR = odds ratio. Sexual orientation, relationship status, current GAHT, and lifetime sex work were excluded from the multivariable model following a backward stepwise selection procedure ($P \leq .20$).
[a]US $1.90 served as the benchmark for extreme poverty, as defined by the World Bank in 2015 at the establishment of the cohort.

(AOR = 0.68; 95% CI = 0.50, 0.92; P = .012). In addition, the analysis revealed that each additional year of age was associated with a slight but statistically significant decrease in the odds of suicidality (AOR = 0.98; 95% CI = 0.97, 1.00; P = .035). Results from an expanded model including year of enrollment are presented in Table B (available as a supplement to the online version of this article at https://ajph.org), which showed no significant association in the multivariable analysis and no change in the main findings. The 5 variables that showed significant associations with suicidality are depicted in Figure 1.

DISCUSSION

In this study, we found a significant association between lifetime discrimination and sexual assault and higher odds of suicidality among TGW in Rio de Janeiro. These findings corroborate existing literature that highlights the detrimental impact of marginalization and violence on mental health across different populations, particularly among transgender, nonbinary, and gender-diverse people.[1,7,14] Our results underscore the need for comprehensive interventions and policy reforms that prioritize the mental health and well-being of this vulnerable population, including those that address discrimination and sexual violence.

Discrimination was significantly associated with higher odds of suicidality, underscoring its pervasive effect on the mental health of Brazilian TGW. This association reflects the broader implications of structural transphobia in Brazil, where systemic discrimination permeates various aspects of life.[1,15] Despite recent advancements in the country, including the Brazilian Supreme Court's criminalization of transphobia as being equivalent to the crime of racism,[16] enforcement remains inconsistent, and many incidents of mistreatment likely

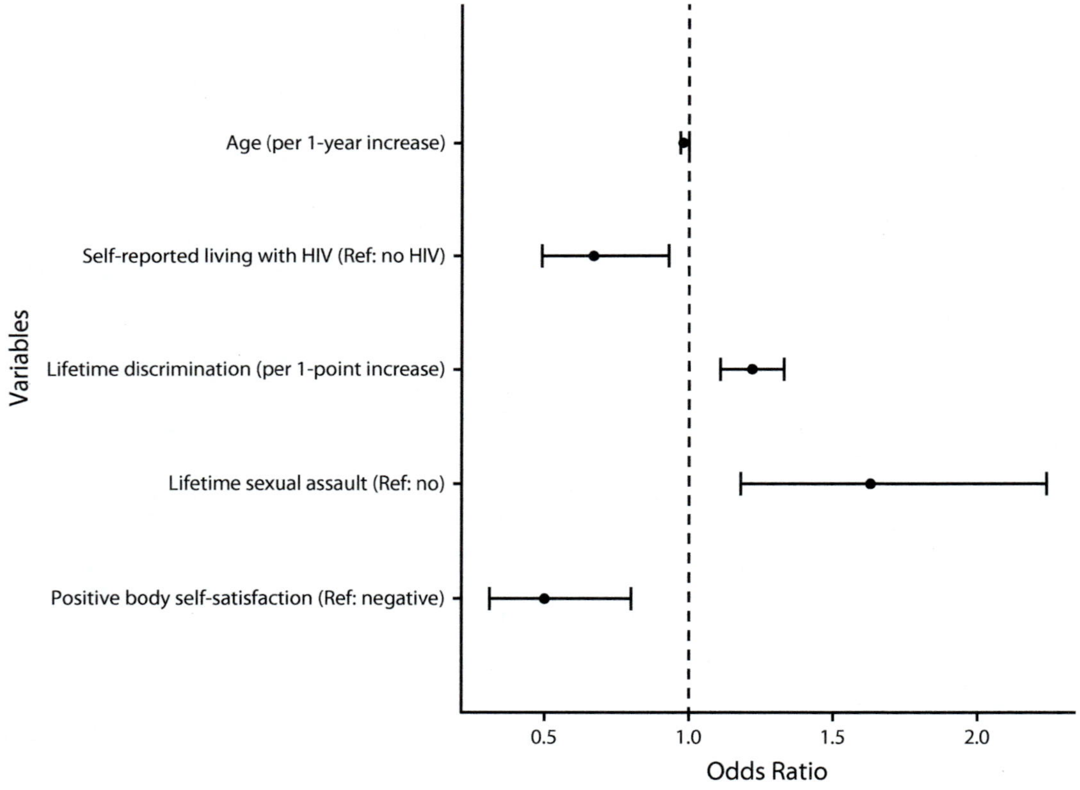

FIGURE 1— Factors Associated With Suicidality Among *Travestis* and Transgender Women in the *Transcendendo* Cohort: Rio de Janeiro, Brazil, 2015–2023

Note. Suicidality was analyzed as an ordinal outcome (no ideation or attempt, ideation only, ideation plus attempt). Variables that were statistically significant in the final multivariable model and are represented in the figure include age (per 1-year increase), self-reported HIV (reference: no HIV), lifetime discrimination (per 1-point increase on a 0–8 scale), lifetime sexual assault (reference: no lifetime sexual assault), positive body self-satisfaction (reference: negative), and positive self-rated health quality (reference: negative). Points represent adjusted odds ratios; horizontal bars indicate 95% confidence intervals; the vertical line denotes odds ratio = 1.

go unreported because of fear of and mistrust in the legal system.[17] Studies have documented a high prevalence of discrimination against TGW in Brazil, with 87.3% to 96% experiencing various forms of exclusion, which are associated with poor mental health outcomes.[1,18–20] These forms of exclusion include barriers to health care access, denial of educational and employment opportunities, social rejection, and harassment in public spaces.[20] Ensuring that victims can safely report incidents and access support services is essential for reducing suicidality and improving the well-being of Brazilian TGW. This need is particularly urgent in the context of rising transphobia in Brazil and worldwide, fueled by the expansion of highly conservative political movements that threaten transgender rights and access to essential services.[21,22]

The relationship between sexual assault and higher odds of suicidality was robust. TGW who experienced lifetime sexual violence had greater odds of more severe levels of suicidality than those who did not have such experiences. Sexual violence can lead to profound psychological trauma, significantly elevating the risk of suicide among survivors.[23] This trauma often results in long-lasting mental health issues such as depression and anxiety, which are known risk factors for suicidality.[24] Previous studies have shown that 40% to 50% of TGW in Brazil experienced lifetime sexual violence, which has been associated with other poor mental health and HIV outcomes.[14,25–27] Another study found that transgender, nonbinary, and gender-diverse people reported experiencing sexual violence at rates up to 25 times more often than heterosexual cisgender men.[28] Our findings underscore the need for culturally responsive support and interventions tailored to TGW victims of sexual violence, especially in highly transphobic settings. Addressing this issue requires training for health care providers, comprehensive violence reporting and response efforts with accompanying legal protections, enforcing existing laws, and ensuring access to trauma-informed care and mental health services.

While physical violence was associated with suicidality in the bivariable model, this association did not remain significant in the multivariable analysis adjusting for covariates and confounders. The prevalence of physical violence in our study was 53.3%, which aligns with previous studies in Brazil,[25,26] emphasizing the need for a holistic approach for addressing the various forms of violence and trauma faced by TGW. Notably, a previous study using data from the *Transcender* cohort (2015–2016) reported significant associations between suicidal behavior and experiences of physical and sexual violence, depression, and other social factors.[9] However, suicidality was analyzed as 2 separate variables (suicidal ideation and suicide attempt) rather than as an ordinal measure, and the study did not find a significant association between discrimination and suicidality, highlighting the additional contribution of our analysis.[9]

Interestingly, positive body self-satisfaction was associated with lower odds of suicidality in our study. This finding underscores the importance of gender-affirming care, as satisfaction with one's body may mitigate some of the negative psychological impacts of gender dysphoria and social stigma. A study found that 85% of transgender men and 50% of transgender women reported significant distress related to gender-related body characteristics, highlighting the widespread impact of body dysphoria on mental health,[29] and previous studies support the role of gender-affirming interventions in improving mental health outcomes among transgender, nonbinary, and gender-diverse people.[30,31] In Brazil, however, access to gender-affirming care, including surgeries, remains limited, with only a few hospitals within SUS offering these services.[15] In addition, significant discrimination and barriers to health care access hinder the provision of comprehensive and necessary gender-affirming care for transgender, nonbinary, and gender-diverse populations.[22] Expanding these services within SUS is essential to ensure that all Brazilian TGW have access to essential medical and psychological support.

HIV status was associated with lower odds of suicidality, potentially suggesting that better access to health care might be implicated in reduced suicide risk. This finding emphasizes the importance of expanding health care access and integrating mental health services within existing health care frameworks for TGW in Rio de Janeiro. In Brazil, people with HIV have their health care needs met by SUS, ensuring they have regular interactions with the health care system. This enables them to access a broad range of services, including mental health care, and such consistent engagement with health care providers may lead to earlier identification and treatment of mental health issues.[32] In addition, those with effectively managed HIV conditions may benefit from specialized HIV care programs that include integrated mental health services, peer support, and counseling, which may further contribute to reducing suicidality.[33]

Finally, an increase in age was associated with lower odds of suicidality, possibly reflecting the development of better coping mechanisms and more stable life conditions over time among Brazilian TGW. Previous studies suggest that older TGW may develop resilience and build stronger social support networks, helping them navigate discrimination and violence and leading to better mental health outcomes.[34] By contrast, younger TGW in Brazil often face more vulnerabilities, including difficulties in accessing health care and poorer HIV and mental health outcomes, such as higher rates of at-risk substance use.[4,35] Thus, policies and programs that include and support TGW across all age groups are needed, especially for younger TGW, fostering resilience and strong social networks throughout their lives to ensure holistic mental health support.

Limitations

This study had limitations. First, the cross-sectional design limits our ability to establish causality. Second, our measures for both exposure and outcome did not capture the frequency or duration of experiences related to discrimination or violence. Third, the reliance on self-reported data introduces the possibility of recall bias. Survivorship bias must also be considered, as we focused on suicidal ideation and suicide attempts, excluding TGW who may have died by suicide. In addition, this was a convenience sample, with initial recruitment through a respondent-driven sampling-based study, followed by open-door enrollment and additional pathways through HIV prevention, care, and related services, which may limit the generalizability of our findings. Although we controlled for self-reported HIV status in our multivariable models, as we considered perceived HIV status to be more directly associated with suicidality outcomes than laboratory-confirmed status, selection bias remains a consideration. However, the inclusion of both people with HIV and those without HIV indicates that the cohort is not restricted by HIV status and captures a broader representation of TGW. Despite these limitations, this study provides, to our knowledge, the first assessment of the association between discrimination, violence, and suicidality among TGW in Rio de Janeiro, using an ordinal measure of suicidality and applying an ideation-to-action framework.[10]

Public Health Implications

Both discrimination and sexual assault were associated with increased suicidality among TGW in Rio de Janeiro. These findings underscore an urgent need for the implementation of antidiscriminatory policies and gender-affirming health care services tailored to the needs of this community. Moreover, the lower odds of suicidality associated with positive body self-satisfaction emphasizes the importance of holistic and inclusive health care interventions. Responsive policies and support systems are necessary to mitigate the high rates of suicidality among Brazilian TGW and to foster a more equitable and supportive environment for this marginalized population. AJPH

ABOUT THE AUTHORS

David R. A. Coelho, Emilia M. Jalil, Biancka Fernandes, Eduardo Peixoto, Thaylla Vianna, Michele Ramos, Cristina M. Jalil, Livia Ferreira, Isabele Barboza Moura, Ruth K. Friedman, Arthur Chaves Araujo, Sandra Cardoso Wagner, Valdiléa G. Veloso, Beatriz Grinsztejn, and Carolina Coutinho are with the Instituto Nacional de Infectologia Evandro Chagas, Fundação Oswaldo Cruz (INI-Fiocruz), Rio de Janeiro, Brazil. Sari L. Reisner is with the Department of Epidemiology, University of Michigan, Ann Arbor. Alex S. Keuroghlian is with the Department of Psychiatry, MaineHealth, Portland.

CORRESPONDENCE

Correspondence should be sent to David R. A. Coelho, MD, MPH, Instituto Nacional de Infectologia Evandro Chagas – Fundação Oswaldo Cruz, Av Brasil, 4365 – Manguinhos, Rio de Janeiro, RJ, 21040-360, Brazil (e-mail: daraujocoelho@mgh.harvard.edu). Reprints can be ordered at https://www.ajph.org by clicking the "Reprints" link.

PUBLICATION INFORMATION

Full Citation: Coelho DRA, Jalil EM, Fernandes B, et al. Association of discrimination and violence with suicidality among *travestis* and transgender women in Rio de Janeiro, Brazil, 2015–2023: a cross-sectional study. *Am J Public Health*. 2026; 116(2):261–269.

Acceptance Date: August 19, 2025.

DOI: https://doi.org/10.2105/AJPH.2025.308280

ORCID iDs:

David R. A. Coelho https://orcid.org/0000-0003-4217-2399

Emilia M. Jalil https://orcid.org/0000-0001-6017-5660

Eduardo Peixoto https://orcid.org/0000-0001-5699-7290

Isabele Barboza Moura https://orcid.org/0000-0002-2435-0254

Sari L. Reisner https://orcid.org/0000-0001-7868-4746

Alex S. Keuroghlian https://orcid.org/0000-0002-6624-8354

Valdiléa G. Veloso https://orcid.org/0000-0002-6622-3165

Beatriz Grinsztejn https://orcid.org/0000-0003-3692-5155

Carolina Coutinho https://orcid.org/0000-0002-9005-8171

CONTRIBUTORS

D. R. A. Coelho, E. Peixoto, V. G. Veloso, B. Grinsztejn, and C. Coutinho conceptualized and designed the study. D. R. A. Coelho, E. Peixoto, and C. Coutinho were involved with data analysis and interpretation. D. R. A. Coelho drafted the original article. E. M. Jalil, B. Fernandes, E. Peixoto, T. Vianna, M. Ramos, C. M. Jalil, L. Ferreira, I. B. Moura, R. K. Friedman, A. C. Araujo, S. C. Wagner, V. G. Veloso, B. Grinsztejn, and C. Coutinho were involved with data acquisition and revised the article draft. S. L. Reisner and A. S. Keuroghlian contributed to revision of the article. V. G. Veloso and B. Grinsztejn acquired the financial support for the project leading to this publication. S. L. Reisner, A. S. Keuroghlian, V. G. Veloso, B. Grinsztejn, and C. Coutinho supervised the study. All authors critically revised the article for important intellectual content, had full access to all the data, and approved the final version for publication.

ACKNOWLEDGMENTS

The *Transcendendo* cohort was supported by funds received by INI-Fiocruz and the Brazilian Ministry of Health. B. Grinsztejn was financed in part by Conselho Nacional de Desenvolvimento Científico e Tecnológico (313265/2023-2) and the Carlos Chagas Filho Foundation for Research Support in the State of Rio de Janeiro (FAPERJ E.26/200.946/2022).

CONFLICTS OF INTEREST

A. S. Keuroghlian declares royalties as editor of a McGraw Hill textbook on transgender and gender-diverse health care and as editor of an American Psychiatric Association textbook on gender-affirming psychiatric care. B. Grinsztejn reports research funding as noted previously.

HUMAN PARTICIPANT PROTECTION

The study was approved by INI-Fiocruz institutional review board. All participants provided written informed consent before participation.

REFERENCES

1. Luz PM, Jalil EM, Castilho J, et al. Association of discrimination, violence, and resilience with depressive symptoms among transgender women in Rio de Janeiro, Brazil: a cross-sectional analysis. *Transgend Health.* 2022;7(1):101–106. https://doi.org/10.1089/trgh.2020.0171
2. Benevides BG, ed. *Dossiê Assassinatos e Violências Contra Travestis e Transexuais Brasileiras em 2021.* Distrito Drag. 2022. Available at: https://antrabrasil.org/wp-content/uploads/2022/01/dossieantra2022-web.pdf. Accessed July 7, 2025.
3. Grinsztejn B, Jalil EM, Monteiro L, Transcender Study Team, et al. Unveiling HIV dynamics among transgender women: a respondent driven sampling study in Rio de Janeiro, Brazil. *Lancet HIV.* 2017;4(4):e169–e176. https://doi.org/10.1016/S2352-3018(17)30015-2
4. Wilson EC, Jalil EM, Moreira RI, et al. High risk and low HIV prevention behaviours in a new generation of young trans women in Brazil. *AIDS Care.* 2021;33(8):997–1001. https://doi.org/10.1080/09540121.2020.1844859
5. *Suicide Worldwide in 2019: Global Health Estimates.* Geneva, Switzerland: World Health Organization; 2021.
6. Kohnepoushi P, Nikouei M, Cheraghi M, et al. Prevalence of suicidal thoughts and attempts in the transgender population of the world: a systematic review and meta-analysis. *Ann Gen Psychiatry.* 2023;22(1):28. https://doi.org/10.1186/s12991-023-00460-3
7. Coimbra BM, Hoeboer CM, Yik J, Mello AF, Mello MF, Olff M. Meta-analysis of the effect of racial discrimination on suicidality. *SSM Popul Health.* 2022;20:101283. https://doi.org/10.1016/j.ssmph.2022.101283
8. Sawyer PJ, Major B, Casad BJ, Townsend SSM, Mendes WB. Discrimination and the stress response: psychological and physiological consequences of anticipating prejudice in interethnic interactions. *Am J Public Health.* 2012;102(5):1020–1026. https://doi.org/10.2105/AJPH.2011.300620
9. Rafael R D MR, Jalil EM, Luz PM, et al. Prevalence and factors associated with suicidal behavior among trans women in Rio de Janeiro, Brazil. *PLoS One.* 2021;16(10):e0259074. https://doi.org/10.1371/journal.pone.0259074
10. Klonsky ED, Saffer BY, Bryan CJ. Ideation-to-action theories of suicide: a conceptual and empirical update. *Curr Opin Psychol.* 2018;22:38–43. https://doi.org/10.1016/j.copsyc.2017.07.020
11. Goldenberg M. The gender of transvestites: the body and sexuality in Brazilian culture [in Portuguese]. *Hist Cienc Saude Manguinhos.* 2009;16(4):1115–1119. https://doi.org/10.1590/s0104-59702009000400015
12. Instituto Brasileiro de Geografia e Estatística. 2022 Census: results. 2024. Available at: https://www.ibge.gov.br/en/statistics/full-list-statistics.html. Accessed July 7, 2025.
13. Chowdhury MZI, Turin TC. Variable selection strategies and its importance in clinical prediction modelling. *Fam Med Community Health.* 2020;8(1):e000262. https://doi.org/10.1136/fmch-2019-000262
14. Reis A, Sperandei S, de Carvalho PGC, et al. A cross-sectional study of mental health and suicidality among trans women in São Paulo, Brazil. *BMC Psychiatry.* 2021;21(1):557. https://doi.org/10.1186/s12888-021-03557-9
15. de Lima RRT, Flor TBM, Noro LRA. Systematic review on health care for transvestites and transsexuals in Brazil. *Rev Saude Publica.* 2023;57:19. https://doi.org/10.11606/s1518-8787.2023057004693
16. de Mello Côrtes A, Gonçalves Buzolin L. Paths towards LGBT rights recognition in Brazil. *Sex Res Soc Policy.* 2024;21(3):1206–1219. https://doi.org/10.1007/s13178-023-00931-y
17. Malta M, Cardoso R, Montenegro L, et al. Sexual and gender minorities rights in Latin America and the Caribbean: a multi-country evaluation. *BMC Int Health Hum Rights.* 2019;19(1):31. https://doi.org/10.1186/s12914-019-0217-3
18. Leite BO, de Medeiros DS, Magno L, et al. Association between gender-based discrimination and medical visits and HIV testing in a large sample of transgender women in northeast Brazil. *Int J Equity Health.* 2021;20(1):199. https://doi.org/10.1186/s12939-021-01541-z
19. Gomes de Jesus J, Belden CM, Huynh HV, et al. Mental health and challenges of transgender women: a qualitative study in Brazil and India. *Int J Transgend Health.* 2020;21(4):418–430. https://doi.org/10.1080/26895269.2020.1761923
20. Lobato MI, Soll BM, Brandelli Costa A, et al. Psychological distress among transgender people in Brazil: frequency, intensity and social causation—an *ICD-11* field study. *Braz J Psychiatry.* 2019;41(4):310–315. https://doi.org/10.1590/1516-4446-2018-0052
21. Coelho DRA, Chen AL, Keuroghlian AS. Advancing transgender health amid rising policy threats. *N Engl J Med.* 2025;392(11):1041–1044. https://doi.org/10.1056/NEJMp2416382
22. Coelho DRA, Ferreira ALN, Vieira WF, Keuroghlian AS, Reisner SL. Mental health outcomes among *travestis* and transgender women in Brazil: a literature review and a call to action for public health policies. *Int J Environ Res Public Health.* 2025;22(7):977. https://doi.org/10.3390/ijerph22070977
23. Bedford CE, Trotter AM, Potter M, Schmidt NB. Minority stress and mental health in lesbian, gay, bisexual, transgender, and queer survivors of sexual assault. *J Trauma Stress.* 2023;36(6):1031–1043. https://doi.org/10.1002/jts.22970
24. Turgumbayev M, Shopabayev B, Dzhansarayeva R, Izbassova A, Beaver K. An examination of associations between sexual assault and health problems, depression or suicidal ideation in a large nationally representative cohort of male and female 20–30-year-olds. *Crim Behav Ment Health.* 2023;33(3):196–212. https://doi.org/10.1002/cbm.2280
25. de Sousa Mascena Veras MA, Menezes NP, Mocello AR, et al. Correlation between gender-based violence and poor treatment outcomes among transgender women living with HIV in Brazil. *BMC Public Health.* 2024;24(1):791. https://doi.org/10.1186/s12889-024-18224-3
26. Ryngelblum M, Grangeiro A, Zucchi EM, et al. Violence, discrimination, and sexual health practices among adolescent men who have sex with men, transgender women and *travestis* in three cities in Brazil. *Cad Saude Publica.* 2023;39(suppl 1):e00142922. https://doi.org/10.1590/0102-311XEN142922
27. dos Santos PMR, dos Santos KC, Magalhães LS, et al. *Travestis* and transsexual women: who are at higher risk for sexually transmitted infections? *Rev Bras Epidemiol.* 2021;24:e210017. https://doi.org/10.1590/1980-549720210017
28. Spizzirri G, Eufrásio RÁ, Abdo CHN, Lima MCP. Proportion of ALGBT adult Brazilians, sociodemographic characteristics, and self-reported violence. *Sci Rep.* 2022;12(1):11176. https://doi.org/10.1038/s41598-022-15103-y
29. Spizzirri G, Eufrásio R, Lima MCP, et al. Proportion of people identified as transgender and non-binary gender in Brazil. *Sci Rep.* 2021;11(1):2240. https://doi.org/10.1038/s41598-021-81411-4
30. Almazan AN, Keuroghlian AS. Association between gender-affirming surgeries and mental health outcomes. *JAMA Surg.* 2021;156(7):611–618. https://doi.org/10.1001/jamasurg.2021.0952
31. Turban JL, King D, Kobe J, Reisner SL, Keuroghlian AS. Access to gender-affirming hormones during adolescence and mental health outcomes among transgender adults. *PLoS One.* 2022;17(1):e0261039. https://doi.org/10.1371/journal.pone.0261039
32. da Rocha ABM, Barros C, Generoso IP, Bastos FI, Veras MA. HIV continuum of care among trans women and *travestis* living in São Paulo, Brazil. *Rev Saude Publica.* 2020;54:118. https://doi.org/10.11606/s1518-8787.2020054002374
33. Alves AM, dos Santos AC, Kumow A, Sato APS, Helena ET D S, Nemes MIB. Beyond access to medication: the role of SUS and the characteristics of HIV care in Brazil. *Rev Saude Publica.* 2023;57:26. https://doi.org/10.11606/s1518-8787.2023057004476
34. Witten TM. It's not all darkness: robustness, resilience, and successful transgender aging. *LGBT Health.* 2014;1(1):24–33. https://doi.org/10.1089/lgbt.2013.0017
35. da Silva RG, de Abreu PD, de Araújo EC, et al. Vulnerability in the health of young transgender women living with HIV/AIDS. *Rev Bras Enferm.* 2020;73(5):e20190046. https://doi.org/10.1590/0034-7167-2019-0046

Political Boundaries, Health Care Gaps: The Link Between Gerrymandering and Federally Qualified Health Center Availability

Auden E. Cote-L'Heureux, BS, and David L. Chin, PhD

See also Lee and Cole, p. 168.

Objectives. To examine how gerrymandering affects federally qualified health center (FQHC) availability in North Carolina.

Methods. We used data from 2004 to 2022 and spatial regression models to correlate gerrymandering metrics with FQHC availability and utilization at the zip code level.

Results. Gerrymandering severity is inversely associated with FQHC availability and utilization. For example, individuals in communities split evenly between 2 state senate districts in this 18-year period (from the end of 2004 through 2022) traveled about 30% farther to their nearest FQHC in 2022 than individuals in communities entirely within a district, and they were up to 20% less likely to visit an FQHC. Increased electoral competitiveness also reduced FQHC availability and utilization. Residential segregation was not linked to FQHC availability or gerrymandering severity.

Conclusions. Gerrymandering weakens local political representation and may lead to reduced access to vital health care services—a structural issue with far-reaching implications for health equity and national policy reform. (*Am J Public Health*. 2026;116(2):270–277. https://doi.org/10.2105/AJPH.2025.308284)

AJPH February 2026, Vol. 116, No. 2

Political determinants of health are most clearly exemplified by specific health-related policy decisions or failures in the distribution of resources, but public health is also linked to political representation. For example, civic engagement correlates positively with health,[1,2] and areas that show large differences in voter participation between age and racial groups report poorer health than areas in which these groups participate at similar levels.[3,4] One barrier to political representation is the gerrymandering of electoral districts, whereby district boundaries are manipulated to favor a political, racial, or other group. Gerrymandering usually "cracks" a cohesively voting community between multiple districts to dilute its voting power or "packs" it into a small number of districts to limit the number of elections it can influence, although the diverse nature of political groups adds complexity.[5] As redistricting in most US states is done by state legislatures, inequitable redistricting is often at the expense of the potential voters with the least political power, who are disproportionately low income and minorities.[6]

Federally qualified health center (FQHC) service sites serve medically underresourced populations throughout the United States, providing health care regardless of a patient's ability to pay. FQHCs depend heavily on government funding, such as special Medicaid reimbursements and Health Resources and Services Administration grants and therefore may be more likely to be directly affected by political dynamics than privately operated institutions.[7] Geographic access to FQHCs has expanded dramatically since their inception in the 1960s, especially since the passage of the Affordable Care Act in 2010 (Pub L No. 111-148, 124 Stat. 855).[8,9]

Past work connecting political representation to public health has been limited yet has yielded striking results;

for example, the implementation of the 1965 Voting Rights Act (Pub L No. 89–110, 79 Stat. 437) in the Southern United States was recently linked to a decrease in infant deaths at the county level over a period of several decades.[10] The impact of inequitable redistricting is less understood. One study inferred from congressional district (CD) shapes that more gerrymandered districts are less exposed to environmental pollution from superfund sites,[11] and highly politicized topics in medicine, such as abortion access, have also been discussed in the context of gerrymandering and minority rule.[12]

We investigated the connection between local political representation and FQHC availability. We built on recent work in the development of local gerrymandering metrics[13,14] and found that the degree of local gerrymandering exhibits an inverse association with FQHC availability and patient volume at the zip code level in the period 2004 to 2022. We focused on North Carolina because it has been the setting for many of the precedent-setting judicial conflicts that are highly salient in political and judicial discussions of redistricting, including *Thornburg v Gingles* (478 US 30 [1986]), *Shaw v Reno* (509 US 630 [1993]), *Rucho v Common Cause* (588 US 684 [2019]), and *Moore v Harper* (600 US 1 [2023]), and because of the availability of voter registration data. We also investigated the correlation of residential segregation as well as electoral competitiveness and representative turnover with FQHC availability.

METHODS

We detail the data sources, define key variables, and describe the metrics calculated for analysis.

Data and Measures

We obtained publicly available individual-level voter registration snapshots and precinct-level shapefiles from the North Carolina State Board of Elections website for the dates October 20, 2006; November 6, 2012; November 6, 2018; and January 1, 2024. Of the 824 total zip code tabulation areas (ZCTAs) in North Carolina, 117 ZCTAs are missing because of unreported precinct-level voter registration data for some counties. These missing ZCTAs differ from the 707 ZCTAs included in the analyses across several key characteristics (Appendix, available as a supplement to the online version of this article at https://www.ajph.org). We obtained decennial census data (2000, 2010, and 2020) and American Community Survey 5-year estimates (2008–2012, 2013–2017, and 2018–2022) at the census block and ZCTA levels from the Integrated Public Use Microdata Series National Historical Geographic Information System.[15] FQHC location and patient volume, as well as medically underserved area designations, are from the Health Resources and Services Administration Uniform Data System.

To test the ZCTA-level effect of gerrymandering on health resource availability and utilization, we used 2 distinct metrics of local gerrymandering: voter dislocation and uncertainty of district membership (UDM). We calculated each metric by grouping individuals by political party (Democratic or Republican) and by race (White or non-White). We excluded individuals not affiliated with a political party from the partisan analyses and individuals without a race designation from the race-based analyses. We calculated all metrics at the census block level and used a population-weighted average to obtain estimates at the level of ZCTAs as designated in 2022 (Appendix).

Voter dislocation is a generalization of the recently developed "partisan dislocation" (D_{party}) metric.[13] This metric measured the degree to which the population of an individual's electoral district represents that individual's geographically nearest neighbors. D_{party} measured the degree to which Democratic and Republican registered voters are dislocated from voters aligned with their political party, and racial voter dislocation (D_{race}) measured the degree to which non-White voters are dislocated from other non-White voters.

UDM measured the degree to which a local community (defined here as all individuals in census blocks with a centroid within a 5-km radius) was split between electoral districts.[14] Under this schema, a community that lay entirely in a single electoral district had a UDM value of 0, a town whose population was split evenly between 2 districts had a UDM value of 1, a town split evenly between 3 districts had a UDM value of about 1.6, and so on. Partisan UDM (UDM_{party}) measured the degree to which Democratic-registered voters were split by district boundaries within a 5-kilometer radius; similarly, racial UDM (UDM_{race}) measured the degree to which non-White voters were split.

We used 2 metrics of electoral competitiveness: (1) vote entropy, which measured how close elections were; and (2) representative turnover, the number of times that the representative of a district changed between 2004 and 2022 as designated in the North Carolina State Board of Elections data set. The entropy metric had shortcomings but was easier to interpret than more complicated metrics[16] (Appendix). We used only general elections that took place in November and manually

AJPH February 2026, Vol. 116, No. 2

curated the vote results data to merge duplicate candidate names. When a ZCTA was split between multiple districts, we calculated the competitiveness and turnover values as a population-weighted average of its constituent district parts.

Statistical Analyses

We measured the association between gerrymandering and change in FQHC availability using a 2-part hurdle regression model with a logistic regression (logit) component that measured the odds of a ZCTA gaining any FQHCs between 2004 and 2022 and a zero-truncated negative binomial (negbin) component that considered the change in FQHC count between 2004 and 2022 in ZCTAs with 1 or more FQHCs.[17] The logit component of the hurdle regression accounted for spatial autocorrelation in FQHC presence by including the total number of FQHCs in all of its neighboring ZCTAs as an exogenous variable (i.e., ZCTAs with shared borders) for each ZCTA. We assessed spatial autocorrelation in the negative binomial model and determined that no spatial correction was required (Appendix Table A; Table 1). In all regression models that included gerrymandering metrics, we used the covariates described earlier plus local gerrymandering, competitiveness, and segregation metrics (Table 1), and we constructed the racial and partisan models separately to avoid biases arising from collinearity. We determined the average for all predictor variables over the 18-year period from 2004 through 2022 to yield a single metric for each ZCTA.

To examine whether the impact on FQHC availability is associated with lower FQHC utilization, we performed linear spatial error regression using the number of individuals per ZCTA who visited any FQHC as the outcome variable. We also built linear spatial error models (SEMs) with the mean distance of non-White residents to their nearest FQHC as the outcome variable.

We tested all models to ensure that the appropriate assumptions were met (Appendix Table A and Figure C), and we

TABLE 1— Population Variables at the Zip Code Tabulation Area (ZCTA) Level: North Carolina, 2004–2022

Variable	Minimum–Maximum	Mean ±SD
Population characteristics		
Population size	231–76 645	13 887 ±14 923
Population density	1.21–2 953.63	180.99 ±325
% Black	0.01–95.6	18.8 ±19.3
% Hispanic/Latino	0.0–47.8	7.5 ±6.7
% Not US citizen	0.00–26.5	3.5 ±3.6
Socioeconomic indicators		
% > 65 y	1.0–57.6	19.1 ±6.7
% rent their home	8.0–99.6	28.3 ±13.3
% own a vehicle	67.7–100	93.8 ±4.4
% have bachelor's degree	2.0–54.9	14.4 ±9.0
% have no health insurance	0.09–73.0	15.0 ±5.9
ZCTA in an MUA		0.89
Income, $	24 536–157 260	46 251 ±16 369
Political and inequality measures		
% Democrat	13–95	54 ±18
% registered to vote	0.05–0.98	0.58 ±0.10
Gini coefficient	0.16–0.63	0.44 ±0.06
Partisan dissimilarity index	0.08–0.22	0.13 ±0.04
Racial dissimilarity index	0.07–0.33	0.15 ±0.08
Vote entropy	0.30–1.07	0.71 ±0.18
Representative turnover	1–6	3.03 ±1.18
Health access variables		
No. of FQHCs	0–12	0.60 ±1.4
% population utilized FQHC	0–75.2	9.8 ±10.6
Congressional district		
D_{party}	0.01–0.24	0.07 ±0.05
D_{race}	0.00–0.29	0.08 ±0.04
UDM_{party}	0.00–0.94	0.19 ±0.22
UDM_{race}	0.00–0.95	0.18 ±0.21
State senate district		
D_{party}	0.00–0.22	0.05 ±0.04
D_{race}	0.00–0.28	0.05 ±0.05
UDM_{party}	0.00–1.43	0.25 ±0.30
UDM_{race}	0.00–1.44	0.24 ±0.28

Note. D_{party} = partisan voter dislocation; D_{race} = racial voter dislocation; FQHC = federally qualified health center; MUA = medically underserved area; UDM_{party} = partisan uncertainty of district membership; UDM_{race} = racial uncertainty of district membership.

did not detect any significant interaction effects in any of the models (Appendix). We conducted statistical analyses using R version 4.4.2 (R Foundation for Statistical Computing, Vienna, Austria).

RESULTS

In 2022, North Carolina contained 824 ZCTAs; of these we obtained gerrymandering measurements for 707 where precinct-level data were available. In 2022, North Carolina housed 459 FQHCs (denoted as FQHCs although distinct from umbrella FQHC organizations, which may operate across multiple states); 405 of these were located within the 707 ZCTAs we analyzed. Table 1 presents ZCTA-level population statistics for the 18-year study period (2004–2022). On average, ZCTAs contained 0.6 FQHCs, with 511 ZCTAs containing 0 FQHCs, 104 only 1 FQHC, and 92 more than 1 FQHC. On average, 926 (9.8%) individuals from each ZCTA visited an FQHC in 2022. Figure 1 shows the statewide distribution of FQHCs in 2022, and Figure 2 shows mean gerrymandering values from 2004 through 2022.

Gerrymandering and Health Center Access

All gerrymandering metrics exhibited a significant inverse association with FQHC availability or utilization at the state senate district (SLDU) or CD level, and none showed a significant positive association (Table 2). In the partisan logit model, UDM_{party} was inversely associated with change in FQHC availability between 2004 and 2022 at the SLDU level, where a community split in half by a district boundary for the entirety of these 18 years was 86% less likely to gain an FQHC during this period than a community that was in a single district. This finding aligns with our observation that although more than 25% of ZCTAs with partisan UDM less than 0.1 contain an FQHC, only 7% of ZCTAs with partisan UDM greater than 1 contain any FQHCs.

We found no significant association between UDM_{party} and FQHC availability at the CD level. D_{party} was inversely associated with change in FQHC availability at the CD level, where a 100% increase in D_{party} corresponded to a 26% decrease in the probability of a ZCTA gaining an FQHC between 2004 and 2022; the relationship was not significant for SLDU-level D_{party}. In the logit model for racial gerrymandering, we obtained nearly identical results for UDM_{race} and D_{race} as we did for UDM_{party} and D_{party}, respectively (Table 2).

Using the negative binomial models, which examined the relationship between local gerrymandering and the change in number of FQHCs (in ZCTAs with at least 1 FQHC), we found that both D_{party} and D_{race} were significantly inversely associated with FQHC availability at the CD level but not at the SLDU level. In this model, a 100% increase in D_{party} (doubling the difference in dislocation between parties) corresponded to 39% fewer FQHCs gained between 2004 and 2022, and a 100% increase in D_{race} corresponded to a 29% decrease.

We found no significant association of UDM with FQHC availability in the negative binomial models (Table 2). We obtained similar results for both the logit and negative binomial statewide models when we used as outcome variables whether a ZCTA contained an FQHC in 2022 and the number of FQHCs per ZCTA in 2022, respectively (rather than the change in FQHC availability between 2004 and 2022; Table 2). An analysis of the change in FQHC availability between 2011 and 2016 as a function of gerrymandering before versus after the 2012 redistricting cycle yielded ambiguous results (Appendix; Figure 2). Patterns in urban versus rural ZCTAs were consistent in directionality but differed in magnitude (Appendix Figure A and Table C).

We found significant correlation between the distance from a non-White individual's residence to their nearest FQHC and both partisan and racial SLDU-level UDM. In both cases, an increase in 1 unit of UDM corresponded to an approximately 30% increase in the distance to the nearest FQHC.

We found a weak but significant correlation between FQHC count and patient volume after adjusting for total population per ZCTA ($R^2 = 0.053$; $P \le .001$). Using SEMs, we analyzed the correlation

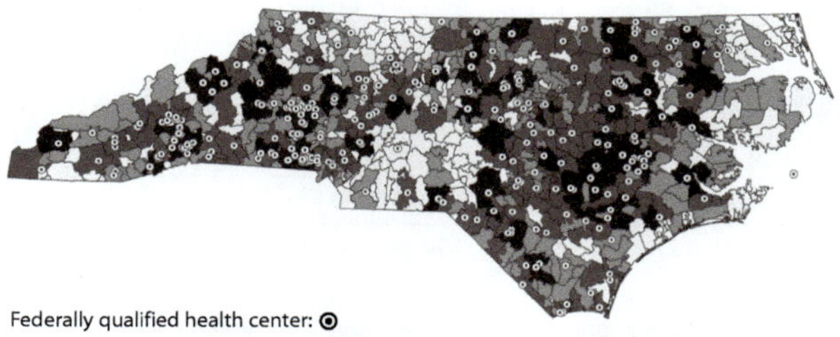

FIGURE 1— FQHC Availability and Patient Volume per ZCTA: North Carolina, 2004–2022

Note. FQHC = federally qualified health center; ZCTA = zip code tabulation area. Black and white points indicate FQHC service sites in operation in 2022. ZCTAs are shaded by total 2022 patient volume.

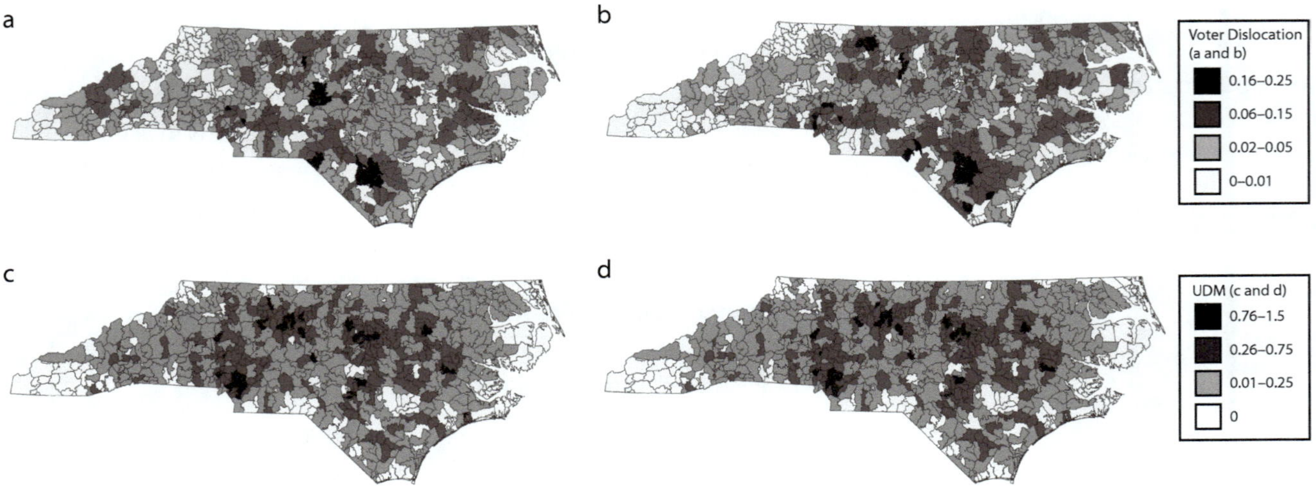

FIGURE 2— Eighteen-Year Aggregate SLDU-Level Gerrymandering Metrics Mapped at the ZCTA Level for (a) Partisan Dislocation, (b) Racial Dislocation, (c) Partisan UDM, and (d) Racial UDM: North Carolina, 2004–2022

Note. SLDU = state senate district; UDM = uncertainty of district membership; ZCTA = zip code tabulation area. In maps of partisan metrics (a and c), darker shades indicate greater partisan bias; in maps of racial metrics (b and d), darker shades indicate greater racial bias. All metrics are given in absolute value. Partisan UDM measures the degree to which the Democratic-affiliated population was split by SLDU boundaries. Racial UDM measures the degree to which the non-White population was split by SLDU boundaries.

between local gerrymandering metrics and the number of patients per ZCTA who visited at least 1 FQHC in 2022 (Table 2). Increases in both partisan and racial UDM were associated with significant decreases in patient volume at the CD level but not the SLDU level. Both D_{party} and D_{race} were inversely associated with patient volume at both the CD and SLDU levels, with a 100% increase in dislocation corresponding to a 13% to 20% decrease in patient volume.

TABLE 2— Estimated Changes in Federally Qualified Health Center Service Site Availability and Patient Volume as a Function of Partisan and Racial Gerrymandering: North Carolina, 2004–2022

FQHC Service Site Metric	Any FQHC in ZCTA,[a] b (95% CI)	No. of FQHCs per ZCTA,[b] b (95% CI)	Distance to FQHC,[c] b (95% CI)	No. of Patients,[d] b (95% CI)
Congressional district				
D_{party}	−0.26 (−0.44, −0.03)	−0.39 (−0.58, −0.11)	0.01 (−0.06, 0.08)	−0.16 (−0.26, −0.04)
D_{race}	−0.29 (−0.42, −0.11)	−0.29 (−0.44, −0.09)	0.05 (−0.02, 0.12)	−0.2 (−0.29, −0.1)
UDM_{party}	0.25 (−0.71, 4.4)	1.26 (−0.61, 12.17)	−0.23 (−0.44, 0.05)	0.42 (−0.21, 1.56)
UDM_{race}	−0.11 (−0.81, 3.1)	0.35 (−0.75, 6.37)	−0.23 (−0.44, 0.07)	0.35 (−0.26, 1.46)
State senate district				
D_{party}	−0.01 (−0.18, 0.2)	0.0 (−0.21, 0.26)	0.02 (−0.02, 0.07)	−0.14 (−0.2, −0.06)
D_{race}	−0.02 (−0.18, 0.17)	−0.08 (−0.26, 0.14)	0.02 (−0.02, 0.07)	−0.13 (−0.19, −0.06)
UDM_{party}	−0.86 (−0.96, −0.49)	−0.85 (−0.98, 0.12)	0.30 (0.03, 0.65)	−0.75 (−0.84, −0.61)
UDM_{race}	−0.86 (−0.96, −0.48)	−0.81 (−0.97, 0.27)	0.34 (0.05, 0.71)	−0.75 (−0.84, −0.61)

Note. CI = confidence interval; D_{party} = partisan voter dislocation; D_{race} = racial voter dislocation; FQHC = federally qualified health center; UDM_{party} = partisan uncertainty of district membership; UDM_{race} = racial uncertainty of district membership; ZCTA = zip code tabulation area. Regression estimates and CIs are expressed as the percentage change in the outcome associated with either a 1-unit increase in the predictor (for UDM) or a 100% increase in the predictor (for voter dislocation).

[a]Logit model measuring the probability that a ZCTA gained an FQHC (2004–2022).

[b]Negative binomial model estimating the number of FQHCs gained per ZCTA (2004–2022).

[c]Spatial error model estimating the mean distance to the nearest FQHC for non-White residents (2022).

[d]Spatial error model estimating the number of patients per ZCTA visiting an FQHC (2022).

Competitiveness and Residential Segregation

In our analysis of electoral competitiveness, we found that increased voter entropy (i.e., greater dispersion of votes among a greater number of candidates) was inversely associated with changes in FQHC availability in the joint logit model and with patient volume in the joint patient volume SEM; both of these models included both partisan and racial gerrymandering metrics as covariates. In the logit model, an increase of 0.1 in 18-year mean vote entropy—approximately the difference in entropy between an election with 2 candidates splitting 50–50 versus an election with a 30–70 split—corresponded to a 14.9% decrease in the probability of a ZCTA containing an FQHC in 2022 (Table 2). In the SEM patient volume model, an increase of 0.1 in mean vote entropy corresponded to a 20.5% decrease in patient volume in 2022. We found no significant correlation between mean entropy and the probability of gaining an FQHC between 2004 and 2022.

In our investigation of residential segregation, simulations of voter clustering by race and political party suggest that residential segregation by race and political party, independent of political boundaries (SLDU or CD), correlates with the respective voter dislocation metrics (Appendix). Therefore, we included 2 metrics of geographic segregation (1 partisan, 1 race based) in our models to control for potential confounding effects. We observed no significant correlation between segregation metrics and our gerrymandering metrics or between segregation metrics and FQHC availability or utilization.

DISCUSSION

Our analyses reveal that areas of North Carolina that were more severely gerrymandered from 2004 to 2022 had smaller increases in FQHC availability in that period and had lower FQHC availability and utilization in 2022. For example, a 1-unit increase in the 18-year average SLDU-level UDM—equivalent to drawing an SLDU border to evenly divide a previously unified community—is associated with a 30% increase in the average distance that a non-White person must travel to their nearest FQHC. Similarly, doubling a ZCTA's CD-level voter dislocation corresponded with an approximately 15% decrease in the likelihood that its residents visited an FQHC.

Although the study design did not permit causal inference, our study extends previous research connecting gerrymandering with dyadic representation by showing that local gerrymandering inversely correlates with health care resource availability.[18–22] Our findings are consistent with the hypothesis that inequitable redistricting has hindered equal access to health care resources at the community level. Our use of a spatial regression model is an advancement on recent research that measured FQHC availability as a function of social determinants of health, which often neglects spatial autocorrelation.[23,24] To our knowledge, this study is the first to employ recently developed local metrics of gerrymandering[13,14] and to explicitly relate gerrymandering and health care. Our results emphasize the importance of considering local effects alongside statewide effects of gerrymandering and demonstrate the potential value of quantifying adverse health impacts to inform new strategies for gerrymandering litigation.

We additionally found that electoral competitiveness was inversely related to FQHC availability and utilization. Gerrymandering has been linked to electoral competitiveness, but causal factors are disputed.[25–27] Studies have found that representatives of more competitive CDs are more responsive to their constituents[28] but that the statewide proportion of incumbent representatives, which would be increased by lower electoral competitiveness, positively correlates with transfers of funds from states to counties.[18]

We found no significant relationship of residential (racial or partisan) segregation with FQHC utilization or gerrymandering. Previous work on the relationship between residential segregation and FQHC availability has been equivocal: 1 nationwide study found a positive correlation,[23] whereas another found no significant trend.[29] Similarly complicated results appear when considering primary care access as a function of residential segregation.[30]

Possible Mechanisms and Implications for Policymakers

Our study design did not permit causal inferences regarding the effect of political representation on health care access. Indeed, some studies suggest that the effect could be in the opposite direction and that excess mortality among minorities reduces their ability to advocate for themselves politically.[31] Nonetheless, the negative association between FQHC availability and long-term UDM may reflect the well-established pattern that splitting communities decreases civic engagement and political awareness.[20–22] Studies have found that residents of a ZCTA split by a CD are less likely to recognize their representative[21] and that misalignment between county borders and state legislative districts corresponds with reduced state to county funding transfers.[18] Similarly, in 2004, communities split by CDs received less federal aid.[19] Because federal funding is essential to founding and maintaining FQHCs,[32] these findings suggest a plausible mechanism. Policies aimed at preventing the fragmentation of communities or ensuring equitable communication between representatives and constituents may make FQHC access more equitable. The significant inverse association between partisan gerrymandering and health care access underscores the potential benefit of delegating redistricting decisions to nonpartisan bodies.

We observed that SLDU-level UDM was more likely to correlate significantly with FQHC access than CD-level UDM, whereas the opposite is true for voter dislocation. This suggests that policy preventing the splitting of communities should focus on SLDU boundaries, although dislocation from one's political group at the CD level may still be problematic.

We also observed that electoral competitiveness was inversely associated with FQHC availability and utilization. These results may be explained by increased representative turnover resulting in lower dyadic representation, but we did not see a significant relationship between turnover and FQHC availability or utilization. Regardless, policies that reduce the dependence of critical health care on electoral dynamics could increase the stability of health care access.

Limitations

Our grouping of individuals by race and political party introduced limitations to our study. We defined racial gerrymandering in reference to the non-White population, recognizing that combining diverse minority groups into a single category was an imperfect approach, particularly in light of the ruling in *Petteway v Galveston County* (86 F.4th 1146 [2024]) that Section 2 of the Voting Rights Act does not apply to such coalitions. Also, because we used separate models to analyze racial and partisan gerrymandering, we could not determine whether the observed effects were predominantly partisan or racial, but the distinction is important because partisan gerrymandering is largely considered nonjusticiable in federal courts, whereas racial gerrymandering remains a violation of federal law.[33] Furthermore, the fact that we excluded unaffiliated voters from our calculations of partisan gerrymandering and used voter registration data rather than actual vote results means that our partisan gerrymandering metrics were only an estimate of the actual effect of inequitable redistricting[5] (Appendix).

Additionally, because of data restrictions, we had to exclude 117 ZCTAs from our analysis; these ZCTAs are biased in terms of several important covariates (Appendix), and inclusion of these ZCTAs for statewide estimates could have given different results.

Lastly, our definition of a community in the UDM calculation as all census blocks within a 5-kilometer radius and our choice to aggregate all predictor and outcome variables at the ZCTA level likely obscured more precise estimates of community boundaries.

Unanswered Questions and Future Research

Further inquiry into how redistricting shapes community health should, in addition to addressing the limitations we have mentioned, examine the effects of local gerrymandering on actual individual or population-level health outcomes, such as mortality, and link local gerrymandering metrics more directly to health-funding allocation, such as intergovernmental transfers of Medicaid funds. These lines of investigation raise important questions about the relative influence of district- or statewide versus community-level factors as well as the effect on health outcomes of redistricting strategies, such as creating majority–minority districts. Policies that reduce the reliance of health care on the responsiveness of representatives will be critical to ensuring more equitable health care provision in an evolving political landscape. Working directly with health care delivery stakeholders is crucial to understanding where the relevant failures in communication and resourcing arise. AJPH

ABOUT THE AUTHORS

Auden E. Cote-L'Heureux was with the Department of Mathematics and Statistics, University of Massachusetts Amherst at the time of this study. David L. Chin is with the Department of Health Policy and Management, School of Public Health and Health Sciences, University of Massachusetts Amherst.

CORRESPONDENCE

Correspondence should be sent to Auden Cote-L'Heureux, 331 Arnold House, 715 North Pleasant St, Amherst, MA 01003 (e-mail: acotelheureu@umass.edu). Reprints can be ordered at https://www.ajph.org by clicking the "Reprints" link.

PUBLICATION INFORMATION

Full Citation: Cote-L'Heureux AE, Chin DL. Political boundaries, health care gaps: the link between gerrymandering and federally qualified health center availability. *Am J Public Health*. 2026;116(2): 270–277.

Acceptance Date: August 22, 2025.

DOI: https://doi.org/10.2105/AJPH.2025.308284

ORCID iDs:
Auden E. Cote-L'Heureux https://orcid.org/0000-0001-5793-7695

David L. Chin https://orcid.org/0000-0002-2341-6207

CONTRIBUTORS

A. E. Cote-L'Heureux conducted the methods design and the data acquisition, analysis, and interpretation. D. L. Chin assisted in methods design and data interpretation. Both authors wrote and revised the article, approved the final version of the article for publication, and agree to be accountable for all aspects of the work in ensuring that questions related to the accuracy or integrity of any part of the work are appropriately investigated and resolved.

ACKNOWLEDGMENTS

The authors would like to acknowledge Daryl DeFord, Jesse Rhodes, and Qian Yu for their valuable feedback at various stages of the data analysis process; Regan Scott-Chin for her careful proofreading and criticism; Phillip Syers for his help understanding this study in a legal and judicial context; and the team managing the Unity compute cluster at the University of Massachusetts Amherst.

CONFLICTS OF INTEREST

The authors have no conflicts of interest to disclose.

HUMAN PARTICIPANT PROTECTION

The University of Massachusetts Amherst internal review board determined that this study does not involve human participant research.

REFERENCES

1. Kim S, Yup KC, You MS. Civic participation and self-rated health: a cross-national multi-level analysis using the World Value Survey. *J Prev Med Public Health*. 2015;48(1):18–27. https://doi.org/10.3961/jpmph.14.031
2. Anderson KA, Dabelko-Schoeny HI. Civic engagement for nursing home residents: a call for social work action. *J Gerontol Soc Work*. 2010;53(3):270–282. https://doi.org/10.1080/01634371003648323
3. Blakely T, Kennedy B, Kawachi I. Socioeconomic inequality in voting participation and self-rated health. *Am J Public Health*. 2001;91(1):99–104. https://doi.org/10.2105/AJPH.91.1.99
4. Homan PA, Brown TH. Sick and tired of being excluded: structural racism in disenfranchisement as a threat to population health equity. *Health Aff (Millwood)*. 2022;41(2):219–227. https://doi.org/10.1377/hlthaff.2021.01414
5. Cox AB, Holden RT. Reconsidering racial and partisan gerrymandering. *Univ Chic Law Rev*. 2011;78(2):553.
6. Niven D, Combs BH, Norwood C, Rossiter KE, Solimine ME. The boundaries of confusion: gerrymandering and racial disparities in state house and congressional district line congruity. *Soc Sci Q*. 2022;103(6):1507–1518. https://doi.org/10.1111/ssqu.13213
7. Snowden LR, Michaels E. Racial bias correlates with states having fewer health professional shortage areas and fewer federally qualified community health center sites. *J Racial Ethn Health Disparities*. 2023;10(1):325–333. https://doi.org/10.1007/s40615-021-01223-0
8. Behr CL, Hull P, Hsu J, Newhouse JP, Fung V. Geographic access to federally qualified health centers before and after the Affordable Care Act. *BMC Health Serv Res*. 2022;22(1):385. https://doi.org/10.1186/s12913-022-07685-0
9. Chang CH, Bynum JPW, Lurie JD. Geographic expansion of federally qualified health centers 2007–2014. *J Rural Health*. 2019;35(3):385–394. https://doi.org/10.1111/jrh.12330
10. Rushovich T, Nethery RC, White A, Krieger N. 1965 US Voting Rights Act impact on Black and Black versus White infant death rates in Jim Crow States, 1959–1980 and 2017–2021. *Am J Public Health*. 2024;114(3):300–308. https://doi.org/10.2105/AJPH.2023.307518
11. Kramar DE, Anderson A, Hilfer H, Branden K, Gutrich JJ. A spatially informed analysis of environmental justice: analyzing the effects of gerrymandering and the proximity of minority populations to US superfund sites. *Environ Justice*. 2018;11(1):29–39. https://doi.org/10.1089/env.2017.0031
12. Basmajian AL. Reproductive gerrymandering, bureaucratic violence, and the erosion of abortion access in the United States. *Med Anthropol Q*. 2024;38(2):179–192. https://doi.org/10.1111/maq.12843
13. DeFord DR, Eubank N, Rodden J. Partisan dislocation: a precinct-level measure of representation and gerrymandering. *Polit Anal*. 2022;30(3):403–425. https://doi.org/10.1017/pan.2021.13
14. Chen SJ, Wang SS-H, Grofman B, Ober RF Jr, Barnes KT, Cervas JR. Turning communities of interest into a rigorous standard for fair districting. *Stanford J Civ Rights Civ Liberties*. 2002;18(1):101–189.
15. Schroeder J, Van Riper D, Manson S, et al. *IPUMS National Historical Geographic Information System*. 2025. Available at: https://doi.org/10.18128/D050.V20.0. Accessed August 27, 2025.
16. Chakravarty SR, Mitra M, Mutuswami S, Pal R. On the probability ratio index as a measure of electoral competition. *Palgrave Commun*. 2020;6(1):96. https://doi.org/10.1057/s41599-020-0466-8
17. Farewell VT, Long DL, Tom BDM, Yiu S, Su L. Two-part and related regression models for longitudinal data. *Annu Rev Stat Appl*. 2017;4:283–315. https://doi.org/10.1146/annurev-statistics-060116-054131
18. Stashko A. Crossing the district line: border mismatch and targeted redistribution. *J Polit*. 2025;87(3). In press. https://doi.org/10.1086/736999
19. Bickers KN, Stein RM. Interlocal cooperation and the distribution of federal grant awards. *J Polit*. 2004;66(3):800–822. https://doi.org/10.1111/j.1468-2508.2004.00277.x
20. Niemi RG, Powell LW, Bicknell PL. The effects of congruity between community and district on salience of US House candidates. *Legis Stud Q*. 1986;11(2):187–201. https://doi.org/10.2307/439875
21. Curiel JA, Steelman T. Redistricting out representation: democratic harms in splitting zip codes. *Election Law J Rules Polit Policy*. 2018;17(4):328–353. https://doi.org/10.1089/elj.2018.0528
22. Bowen DC. Boundaries, redistricting criteria, and representation in the US House of Representatives. *Am Polit Res*. 2014;42(5):856–895. https://doi.org/10.1177/1532673X13519127
23. Ko M, Ponce NA. Community residential segregation and the local supply of federally qualified health centers. *Health Serv Res*. 2013;48(1):253–270. https://doi.org/10.1111/j.1475-6773.2012.01444.x
24. Lee EK, Donley G, Ciesielski TH, Freedman DA, Cole MB. Spatial availability of federally qualified health centers and disparities in health services utilization in medically underserved areas. *Soc Sci Med*. 2023;328:116009. https://doi.org/10.1016/j.socscimed.2023.116009
25. Henderson JA, Hamel BT, Goldzimer AM. Gerrymandering incumbency: does nonpartisan redistricting increase electoral competition? *J Polit*. 2018;80(3):1011–1016. https://doi.org/10.1086/697120
26. Forgette R, Garner A, Winkle J. Do redistricting principles and practices affect US state legislative electoral competition? *State Polit Policy Q*. 2009;9(2):151–175. https://doi.org/10.1177/153244000900900202
27. Carson JL, Crespin MH, Eaves CP, Wanless E. Constituency congruency and candidate competition in US House elections. *Legis Stud Q*. 2011;36(3):461–482.
28. Griffin JD. Electoral competition and democratic responsiveness: a defense of the marginality hypothesis. *J Polit*. 2006;68(4):911–921. https://doi.org/10.1111/j.1468-2508.2006.00479.x
29. Abbeele VD, Rees S. Assessing the impact of residential segregation and population composition on the county-level supply of federally qualified health centers. 2022. Available at: https://escholarship.org/uc/item/9gd7194f. Accessed August 27, 2025.
30. Gaskin DJ, Dinwiddie GY, Chan KS, McCleary RR. Residential segregation and the availability of primary care physicians. *Health Serv Res*. 2012;47(6):2353–2376. https://doi.org/10.1111/j.1475-6773.2012.01417.x
31. Rodriguez JM, Geronimus AT, Bound J, Dorling D. Black lives matter: differential mortality and the racial composition of the US electorate, 1970–2004. *Soc Sci Med*. 2015;136–137:193–199. https://doi.org/10.1016/j.socscimed.2015.04.014
32. Wakefield M. Federally qualified health centers and related primary care workforce issues. *JAMA*. 2021;325(12):1145–1146. https://doi.org/10.1001/jama.2021.1964
33. Tofighbakhsh S. Racial gerrymandering after *Rucho v. Common Cause*: untangling race and party. *Colum Law Rev*. 2020;120(7):1885–1928.

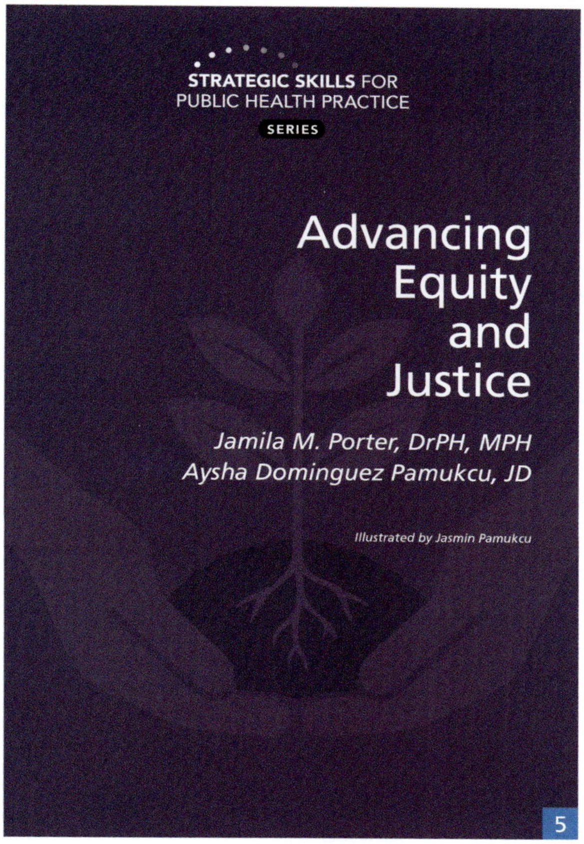

ISBN 978-0-87553-3599, 220 PP., 2026,
SOFTCOVER, PRINT ON DEMAND

Strategic Skills for Public Health Practice: Advancing Equity and Justice

Jamila M. Porter, DrPH, MPH, and Aysha Dominguez Pamukcu, JD

Strategic Skills for Public Health Practice: Advancing Equity and Justice is a call to reimagine public health as a dynamic social movement rooted in community leadership. Grounded in bold vision and practical application, this book confronts the root causes of health inequities — powerful systems that determine how long and how well we live. *Advancing Equity and Justice* challenges practitioners to move beyond limited technical fixes to embrace the moral clarity and collective action necessary to improve health for all.

APHABOOKSTORE.ORG

APHA PRESS

AN IMPRINT OF AMERICAN PUBLIC HEALTH ASSOCIATION